ACCOUNTABILITY
IN NURSING

Six Strategies to Build and
Maintain a Culture of Commitment

Eileen Lavin Dohmann, RN, MBA, NEA-BC

HCPro

Accountability in Nursing: Six Strategies to Build and Maintain a Culture of Commitment is published by HCPro, Inc.

Copyright © 2009 HCPro, Inc.

ISBN 978-1-60146-345-6

HCPro, Inc., provides information resources for the healthcare industry.

HCPro, Inc., is not affiliated in any way with The Joint Commission, which owns the JCAHO and Joint Commission trademarks. MAGNET™, MAGNET RECOGNITION PROGRAM®, and ANCC MAGNET RECOGNITION® are trademarks of the American Nurses Credentialing Center (ANCC). The products and services of HCPro, Inc., and The Greeley Company are neither sponsored nor endorsed by the ANCC. The acronym MRP is not a trademark of HCPro or its parent corporation.

Eileen Lavin Dohmann, RN, MBA, NEA-BC, Author	Audrey Doyle, Copyeditor
Rebecca Hendren, Senior Managing Editor	Liza Banks, Proofreader
Emily Sheahan, Group Publisher	Susan Darbyshire, Art Director
Shane Katz, Cover Designer	Matt Sharpe, Production Supervisor
Janell Lukac, Graphic Artist	Jean St. Pierre, Director of Operations

Advice given is general. Readers should consult professional counsel for specific legal, ethical, or clinical questions.

Arrangements can be made for quantity discounts. For more information, contact:

HCPro, Inc.
P.O. Box 1168
Marblehead, MA 01945
Telephone: 800/650-6787 or 781/639-1872
Fax: 781/639-2982
E-mail: *customerservice@hcpro.com*

Visit HCPro at its World Wide Web sites:
www.hcpro.com and *www.hcmarketplace.com*

3/2009
21646

CONTENTS

Contents

DEDICATION

One of my personal goals has been to be published. Taking on a book as a first published work has been daunting—far more challenging than I ever imagined. Many special people have made this book possible and I am very grateful to all of them.

Mark Hawkins and John Scanlon of Financial Transformations, Inc.: As friends and business colleagues, I have worked with them during the past fifteen-plus years. Our weekly conversations are my "touchstone" to stay focused on what I am trying to accomplish and to always think about how I can be better at what I do. They taught me to understand and live my own leadership story. They challenge me to be and stay on my own journey to professional excellence.

Rebecca Hendren and the great people at HCPro: Their constant support and encouragement helped, especially during the many times I wanted to "throw in the towel." They came up with one creative idea after another to keep me going and to ease the work.

Executive leadership, my peers, and colleagues at Medicorp Health System: They encourage me to grow professionally and be continually challenged. They have allowed me to "develop and practice" my accountability approach and techniques with and on all of them. They have supported my growth and development with opportunities I never could have imagined. Thank you for allowing me to tell our accountability story. I am proud and privileged to work with all of you.

My family: My husband and three sons deal with my long work hours with support and encouragement. They remind me to not take myself too seriously. When one of my ideas sounds a bit wild, they have great ways of grounding me while challenging me to grow personally and professionally. They remind me to have fun at everything I do.

Dedication

My parents: My mother, as a former vice president, nursing, has always been a mentor and role model. She has always challenged me to be the best at what I am, especially as a nurse. To my father, who has always said, " 'I' (Eileen), you can be and do whatever you want. Just put your mind to it. Just do it!"

To all of you, this book is dedicated to you. Thank you all very much!

ABOUT THE AUTHOR

Eileen Lavin Dohmann, RN, MBA, NEA-BC

Eileen Lavin Dohmann, RN, MBA, NEA-BC, is vice president of nursing at Mary Washington Hospital in Fredericksburg, VA. She is responsible for nursing care and services as well as operational oversight for MW Home Health and Hospice and The Cancer Center of Virginia. Her passion at Mary Washington Hospital has been enhancing patient care and service through accountability, focused management, and leadership development of the nursing leaders. With 25 years' experience as a nurse, she is an advocate for the profession of nursing and excellence in nursing practice.

Prior to her roles at Mary Washington Hospital, Dohmann served as administrator for several small and large home health and hospice programs, where she started and led new programs and services.

Dohmann has presented at several national conferences on accountability, management development, and hospice program development. She received her BSN from Fairfield (CT) University, and her MBA from Averett University in Danville, VA.

She lives with her husband in Centreville, VA, and is the proud mom of three young professional and college-aged sons.

HOW TO USE THE TOOLS ON THE CD-ROM

With this book, nurse managers and leaders will learn how to engage people in what they are doing, secure their commitment, and ensure they follow through on their commitments. All of the book's tools and templates can be found on the accompanying CD-ROM. Put your organization's name on the forms, customize them to fit your needs, and print them out for immediate staff use.

Files on the CD-ROM

To adapt any of the files to your own facility, simply follow the instructions below to open the CD. If you have trouble reading the forms, click on "View," and then "Normal." To adapt the forms, save them first to your own hard drive or disk (by clicking "File," then "Save as," and changing the system to your own). Then change the information to fit your facility, and add or delete any items that you wish to change.

The following file names on the CD-ROM correspond with tools listed in the book:

File name	Document
Fig 1-1.rtf	Profound Distinctions
Fig 1-2.rtf	Individual's Attitudes toward Results
Fig 1-3.rtf	Accountability Culture: How We Respond to Attitudes
Fig 2-1.rtf	Accountability Pocket Card—Adaptable Word Version
Fig 2-1.pdf	Accountability Pocket Card—PDF Version
Fig 2-2.pdf	Assessing the Energy in the Room
Fig 2-3.pdf	Net Forward Energy
Fig 3-1.rtf	Accountability Language
Fig 4-1.rtf	How to "be" in a Meeting
Fig 4-2.rtf	Meeting Redesign Tool
Fig 4-3.rtf	Commitment Log

ACCOUNTABILITY IN NURSING

The CD-ROM also includes the following bonus tools not found in the book:

File name	Document
DNA_Tool.rtf	DNA Communication Tool
Effective_questions.rtf	Effective Questions to Ask
Clear_speaker.rtf	Tips for Being a Clear Speaker and an Active Listener
CPR_Tool.rtf	Communication CPR Tool
Agenda.rtf	Agenda Template to Facilitate Productive Meetings

Installation Instructions

This product was designed for the Windows operating system and includes Word files that will run under Windows 95/98 or later. The CD will work on all PCs and most Macintosh systems. To run the files on the CD-ROM, take the following steps:

1. Insert the CD into your CD-ROM drive.

2. Double-click on the "My Computer" icon, next double-click on the CD drive icon.

3. Double-click on the files you wish to open.

4. Adapt the files by moving the cursor over the areas you wish to change, highlighting them, and typing in the new information using Microsoft Word.

5. To save a file to your facility's system, click on "File" and then click on "Save As." Select the location where you wish to save the file and then click on "Save."

6. To print a document, click on "File" and then click on "Print."

INTRODUCTION

Accountability is a word we often hear in conjunction with discussions about leadership. But what does accountability mean? And what do we mean by accountability when we talk about it in relation to nursing?

Accountability is a commitment, a promise to deliver a result by a given time. It is a word we often use in nursing. And just as often, it is a condition we find difficult to establish.

Accountability is a necessary tool if you are looking to achieve excellence, whether as an individual, as a group, or as an organization. Being a leader requires accountability. Walk through a day in the life of a nurse or nurse leader and you will see that accountability permeates everything we do. As nurses and nurse leaders, we continually strive to get people to do things: from the patients we teach about managing their new diagnosis, to nurse managers who are working with their staff to improve Core Measure performance, to the chief nursing officer who is working with senior executives to engage them in a discussion about the value of nursing in an acute care hospital.

Simply put, accountability is about commitments: getting people to commit to doing something and then knowing they will follow through on their commitment. It is always a challenge. What people say they will do can be very different from what they actually do, and what we think they committed to is often worlds apart from what they think they committed to. Yet accountability is critical to being an effective nurse leader.

Nurse leaders need engaged and committed nurses. We need quick, surefire techniques that allow us to engage people in what we are doing, gain their commitments, and ensure that they perform the actions needed to achieve those commitments.

In this book, you will find those surefire techniques so that you can use your time effectively and efficiently; always moving toward excellence through accountability. The book is separated into chapters covering different relationships. You can read the book as a whole, or you can read chapters 1 and 2 and then choose to read chapters on the particular relationships that interest you, such as those with physicians or senior executives. To facilitate ease of use for the reader, some ideas and strategies are explained in each of chapters 3 through 8 so that readers may flip to whichever chapter they prefer.

If you master accountability you will achieve great patient care, great staff morale and performance, great professional fulfillment, and great career success.

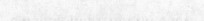

WHAT IS ACCOUNTABILITY?

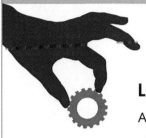

Learning Objectives

After reading this chapter, the participant will be able to:

✓ Differentiate between responsibility and accountability

✓ Describe how accountability is demonstrated

✓ Explain why accountability is important in the nursing profession

Difference Between Accountability and Responsibility

Before you can work toward achieving accountability, you need to ensure that you understand what is meant by the term and the way in which we will be using it in this book. We frequently hear the terms *responsibility* and *accountability* used interchangeably, but they do not mean the same thing.

If you look up dictionary definitions, you'll find the following explanations:

- Accountability:
  - Responsible for something
  - Capable of being explained
- Responsibility:
  - Being accountable for something
  - Authority to make decisions independently

These definitions are not much help. So, let's consider alternative definitions. A powerful distinction can exist between accountability and responsibility.

An effective way to distinguish them is as follows:

- Accountability = A commitment to others to deliver and account for a result by a given date

- Responsibility = An authority over people to have them respond to one's direction

Accountability is about the results to be delivered. A result is a desired situation that can be described. It is measurable, observable, and time-limited, such as "I will have the operating room reorganized by Friday."

Responsibility is about things that will respond to you. Think of responsibility as what is included in a job description. Your job responsibilities include the things you need to do to perform your job, including staffing, budgeting, and so on.

In the next two sections, I will show you the power of these distinctions. It turns out that accountability and responsibility appear in different ways depending on the role you fill. You will encounter accountability and responsibility at work in two ways: through your organizational roles and your interpersonal interactions. You can use these distinctions to better see the game you are playing at any moment in time—and win that game!

Accountability and Organizational Roles

Professionals in any organization often find themselves assuming three different roles at different times: supervisor, manager, and leader. Each is a profoundly different kind of work that calls for different mindsets and skills. The three represent different uses of accountability and responsibility, as shown in Figure 1.1.

FIGURE 1.1: PROFOUND DISTINCTIONS

	Accountable	Not Accountable
Responsible	Manager	Supervisor Professional
Not Responsible	Leader	Observer Worker

A supervisor is responsible and not accountable

As supervisors, we are responsible for a well-defined set of activities to be carried out in a prescribed way. As professionals, we know the work to be done. We can tell someone else what to do and how to do it. However, as a professional, we are not held accountable for another professional's actions and results. For example, a supervisor is responsible for stocking the operating room with supplies in a certain way according to a prescribed inventory, but is not responsible for how the supplies are used or what effects the supplies have.

A manager is accountable and responsible

As a nurse manager, you are responsible for how your unit runs, the staff you employ, and the care that is provided. You have the authority to run your unit, and staff members respond to your direction. In addition, you have to produce results with those resources. The results the nurse manager is accountable for range from patient length of stay to care quality, from nurse productivity to staffing costs. A manager has all of the resources needed to deliver a well-defined set of expected results. Managers organize, oversee, and respond to produce results. A manager needs to influence others to achieve expected results with available resources. It is about realizing expected results rather than performing a certain activity.

A leader is accountable and not responsible

Leadership appears when a person has intent that far exceeds his or her reach. The intent, expressed as a vision or goal, cannot be achieved with the resources for which the person is responsible. A leader envisions exciting possibilities and enlists others in their shared vision. This person has accepted accountability for an outcome that is beyond his or her ability to produce.

This scary situation is easy to resolve . . . in principle. A leader has to reach out to and enroll others who have the necessary responsibility for resources. The leader, by declaring a bold goal, discovers possibilities and opportunities that are hidden. Leadership is about generating commitments from others to produce results that will contribute to the leader's goal.

For example, as a vice president of nursing, I am accountable for the quality of patient care that is provided in our hospital. I know that because when patients or families have a compliment or complaint, they find my office. However, I don't provide one ounce of patient care myself. Furthermore, I am not positioned or informed enough to tell anyone what to do for a particular patient. I do not have responsibility for the care of any patient. Yet I am accountable for the quality of that care. I have to influence many nurses and others to be successful. I have to enroll them in my vision and goal to provide the highest level of quality care to our patients.

When I speak of leadership in this book, I am referring to a role a person has assumed. "Leadership" is not defined by a job title and does not refer to a position of authority. Leadership is a choice a person makes. You cannot delegate leadership or make someone a leader. Individuals define and step into leadership roles.

To perform as a leader, you need to tell your *leadership story*. You need to define what you stand for, and that should be a compelling future with passion, energy, and drama. People will follow a leader because they want to commit to the future the leader stands for; they want to be part of something that is bigger than they are and that involves a state and passion of which they want to be part. People want visions of the future to reflect their own aspirations. A leader makes a declaration of a compelling future that will attract the attention and interest of others.

Designing Organizational Roles and Culture

The differences between a supervisor, a manager, and a leader show up dramatically for me every day with our patient flow coordinators. They are responsible for patient placement and flow from the emergency room and intake to the nursing units. Through our electronic bed board, they receive requests for beds and place patients in those beds. Depending on many variables, such as number of admissions and discharges or staffing, their job can be easy or challenging.

The most frequent complaint that I hear from them is this:

> *"I need help on a particular unit. Every time I try to give them more than one admission at a time, I get pushback. I can't make them accept the patient because they don't report to me."*

In other words, the coordinators do not have authority and the units do not respond to requests. They are saying, "Given my level of responsibility, I am not accountable."

Using Figure 1.1 as a reference, the patient flow coordinator is a "supervisor" who is responsible for the process of patient flow: ensuring that workers follow procedure and protocols regarding patient placement. The results we want from patient flow require the participation of many others, including staff members, nurse managers, transporters, radiology, lab, physicians, and others. If we want coordinators to be accountable for high-performance, high-quality patient flow, they have to assume a leadership role. They need to be able to influence staff and managers on units to assist with effective patient flow and placement. As supervisor, the coordinator is only about telling, checking, and reporting.

As vice president of nursing, I can now see the challenge. What is my intent? Do I make the coordinators managers with responsibility for nursing unit beds and other unit staff members? Or do I ask them to be leaders where they enroll other managers in their campaign for certain patient flow outcomes? Or do I limit them to supervisory roles?

As you might guess, giving them more responsibility (authority) over the other units would create a mess. Yet I want my patient flow coordinators to be more than supervisors. I need them to step into leadership roles. So, how do I get them to accept this new accountability?

Moving beyond a risk-averse culture

As I move through this process, I can expect to run into a culture constraint, and it's important to remember just how large a role culture plays in accountability. Throughout our lives and our professional training, we are taught to keep our promises and our commitments. We are taught to avoid risk. Remember the saying, "Don't commit to things you cannot deliver"? Therefore, our instinct is to be accountable for results only when we have the responsibilities needed to deliver. The de facto culture in most organizations is "avoid accountability that exceeds my domain of responsibility." And often it is even more risk-averse than that: "Define my responsibility so narrowly that there is no significant outcome that I can be held accountable for."

It turns out that in medicine and healthcare delivery, almost all the desired outcomes call for professionals to be ready to move beyond supervisory roles and into management and leadership roles. That means we cannot live with the de facto risk-averse culture. We have to create an accountability culture!

Interpersonal Interactions in an Accountability Culture

Accountability is a choice people make. Sometimes the choice is tied to a job. Nursing unit managers in our hospital agree to be accountable for certain outcomes. Often the choice is a decision in response to an opportunity or a request. You can give responsibility to a person, but you cannot give accountability. The person has to choose it. You can request it, but you cannot order it. Accountability is a choice.

To have a culture that promotes accountability, we need a culture that encourages and celebrates people making choices. We need a culture that celebrates success. We must promote a culture that celebrates the learning that occurs when we don't succeed.

In an accountability culture, there is no punishment. Punishment causes people to be risk-averse and avoid accountability. Instead, an accountability culture promotes learning, performing, and improving. What does accountability look like in such a culture?

With accountability you are seeking a result. You need someone to be accountable for the result. Imagine you are asking a person to accept accountability as either a manager or a leader. Over time, you will find that the person will either be accountable or not be accountable. We shall see later that it is often difficult up-front to tell how they will respond. At some point, the resultant situation will be examined and either there will be a result or there will not be a result. Figures 1.2 and 1.3 show how all of this appears in an accountability culture.

You may experience four situations that represent attitudes the person can take regarding the desired result. All four could be acceptable in a de facto culture. Only two are acceptable in an accountability culture.

FIGURE 1.2: INDIVIDUALS' ATTITUDES TOWARD RESULTS

	Not Accountable	Accountable
No Results	Individual #1: Reward effort	Individual #3: Learning
Results	Individual #2: Not predicted, no control, luck	Individual #4: Performing

---

You may encounter individual #1 who is not accountable and is not achieving results. This is the staff nurse whom you counsel for time and attendance issues. Her response:

> *"I know I have to do better with being on time. At least I don't cause you any trouble. I have a good attitude and my patients like me, not like some of the other folks on our floor. You should be talking to them. I'll try to do better with being on time."*

This staff person wants to be rewarded for a good effort.

Individual #2 is not accountable and is getting the desired results. This is the manager who is achieving his or her patient satisfaction goal this month and whom you approach to understand what attributed to this month's success. The manager's response:

> "I have no idea. I do the same things each month and one month the scores are low and the next month they are high."

Producing the desired result is an accident, a matter of luck. No one knows what will happen next month. The manager does not appear to have control over the results.

Individual #3 is being accountable and is not achieving the desired results. This is the manager who has not achieved his or her Core Measures performance in the past two months. You approach the manager, who responds:

> "I know we aren't performing where we should. I own these scores. I have reviewed the performance with the quality data abstractors and we will be doing three things differently this month. I'll be able to monitor our progress each week because my secretary will be auditing every discharged chart."

This manager owns the results and is learning how to best improve performance. She is being accountable.

The last individual, #4, is accountable and is achieving the desired results. This is the manager who is consistently hitting budgeted productivity performance targets. When you discuss results with the manager, he or she can tell you exactly what is being done in terms of productivity and can predict the level of productivity for the current period.

When you encounter each of these individuals, how do you respond in an accountability culture? Figure 1.3 summarizes the responses.

FIGURE 1.3: ACCOUNTABILITY CULTURE: HOW WE RESPOND TO ATTITUDES

	Not Accountable	Accountable
No Results	Individual #1: Unacceptable (call it)	Individual #3: Investing for future results
Results	Individual #2: Unacceptable (call it)	Individual #4: Celebration, model

---

For the individual who is not accountable and is not achieving results (#1), you need to identify the behavior/performance as unacceptable and "call it" as such. What is unacceptable is that this individual has accepted a position and rejected the accountability that comes with it. Now this individual is using "effort" as an excuse for not performing and for not committing to fixing the nonperformance.

The individual who is not accountable and is achieving results (#2) is also demonstrating unacceptable behavior that needs to be "called." There is no learning and no commitment for maintaining performance.

An accountability culture does not reward effort. It does not reward luck. Accountability rewards commitment and results.

For #3, the individual who is accountable and is not yet achieving results, you should invest in the idea of learning in order to obtain future results. But you also need to set realistic limits on how long you can wait for these results. As long as this manager is continually learning and improving, you reward the behavior and invest in the future.

The manager who is accountable and is achieving results (#4) is someone you want to celebrate and reward. You also want to model the manager's practices and use him or her as a teacher.

These are the individuals who should receive 80% of your time and attention. Too often, we spend 80% of our time on the individuals who are in the first two categories.

In an accountability culture, a manager is expected to express accountability. In effect, the manager wears a button on his or her shirt that says: "Ask me what I am accountable for." In an accountability culture, individuals are encouraged and expected to assume leadership roles. To get this kind of behavior you have to avoid punishment downstream . . . and be very good at establishing accountability upstream.

You want to avoid the downstream conversation about "unacceptable" attitude. Fortunately, there are tools you can master to be effective in establishing accountability and to have productive meetings.

You need to step beyond your responsibilities, as leadership appears when a person has intent that far exceeds his or her reach. The intent, expressed as a vision or a goal, cannot be achieved with the resources the person is responsible for. Therefore, a leader has to enroll others with different responsibilities. Leadership efforts hold the promise of extraordinary results.

Accountability is the tool to use to achieve excellence in leadership. The next chapter discusses the tools you can use to promote accountability.

ACCOUNTABILITY TOOLS

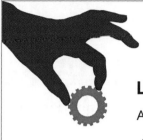

Learning Objectives

After reading this chapter, the participant will be able to:

✓ List the six tools in accountability

✓ Explain the six tools for holding oneself and others accountable

Everything You Need to Hold Yourself and Others Accountable

Now that you understand what accountability looks and sounds like, how do you become accountable and get accountability from those you encounter? In this chapter, you will learn about quick, surefire techniques that will allow you to do each of the following:

- Engage people in what you are doing

- Gain their commitments

- Have them act to achieve those commitments

You will find techniques that will allow you to use your time effectively and efficiently; always in action toward achieving excellence through accountability.

The good news is that the techniques, for the most part, involve activities with which you are already familiar. Even more good news is that, because they are familiar, others will recognize and accept them. And even further good news is that you have opportunities every day to try them out and further develop them so that they become good habits.

Examine your style

Let's talk about your style. That's the way you make things happen and get things done. This chapter will show you how to develop your style so that it generates accountability. We will talk about using that style to make the meetings you are in productive. Everyone's time is limited, so it pays to be effective in meetings and to attend meetings that are productive.

Style is something that is personal to you, but most likely you don't think about it. It is on autopilot. You walk into a room and, depending on whether it's your meeting or someone else's, you fall into a rote behavior.

You need to change that. Be self-conscious about your style as a manager, as a leader.

The techniques in this book were intentionally developed over the years. I sought out people who were interested in executive productivity and leadership, and they helped me to craft and test ideas as I built up a set of tools that had power.

My partners in this were Mark Hawkins and John Scanlon, who also contributed to this book. A lot of the ideas came from work done by Dennis Wagner and Doug Krug, and my own organization has a leadership program that helped to shape my thinking. As you develop your leadership and management style, put together your own learning group. Steal shamelessly and test frequently.

This chapter should be part of your journey toward developing a powerful style. The chapter also discusses two types of tools: One type is a way of speaking; the other a way to have productive meetings.

Six Accountability Language Tools

As we grow into supervisor, manager, and leadership roles, many of us find that most of our work happens in meetings and that work always involves speaking.

Over my career in several organizations, I have observed that most meetings do not lead to clear commitments and accountability. They are informational. Opinions and assessments are common and there is a lot of idle chatter.

This is not the defining work of managers or executives. If you are a manager or executive and you find yourself in these information exchange meetings, you are not doing executive, high-level work. The work of executives and managers is to generate commitments, make commitments, and deliver on commitments.

Think about that meeting you have been in where you are working on a problem. During the meeting, everyone agrees to the plan. You see heads nodding, and people smiling and looking engaged. Six months later, you are in the same meeting, fixing the same problem again. What happened? It turns out that six months earlier there were no commitments; no one accepted accountability. To leave a meeting with accountability in place you have to use speech acts that create the energy, content, and conditions for accountability to take place.

This chapter presents six tools to use to have productive meetings. They are an accountability language for you to learn; a new way of speaking. The words we use can either dampen accountability or trigger accountability. The next time you encounter a situation where you want to achieve accountability, try using language that produces accountability.

I have found the following speech acts to be very effective:

1. **Framing:** Turn on the listening you need

2. **Effective questions:** Turn on the creative power of the participants

3. **Active listening:** Make sure people are being heard and understood

4. **Requests and offers:** Generate commitments

5. **Hear yes/no:** Verify accountability

6. **Acknowledgment:** Celebrate behavior that works

These words create the necessary conditions. Each one creates a positive dynamic that makes it easy for accountability to happen.

1. Framing

Framing is when you ask the audience to listen and process what they are hearing in a positive way. It creates the listening environment in which you can speak. It creates one common mindset in the room and enables participants to do the correct work.

If six people are in the room, you have six mindsets and six kinds of listening. Remember, most people will be on autopilot. They will be operating from habit.

It is possible that in the room the following people will be listening:

- Person A: How will I respond to those urgent e-mails when I get back to my office?

- Person B: What critical assessment can I make of what is being said in order to look smart?

- Person C: What can I do to not be noticed, to not get an assignment?

- Person D: That's interesting, that reminds me of the time . . .

- Person E: I wonder who made her slides.

- Person F: How will her proposal disrupt my operations, my plans?

This does not bode well for a productive meeting. And this is natural; no one is being intentionally uncooperative.

It is easy to fix the random mindset in the room by asking people to be a certain way, to do a specific kind of work, and to be open to the possibility of accountability. This is what framing sounds like:

- I ask that all of us be in our leadership role for this session
- I ask that we work toward our vision of a high-quality nursing care program in nine months
- I ask that everybody listen to the presentation to discern opportunities we can pursue to make progress toward our goal
- Please be prepared to make commitments at the end, thank you

Everyone wants to do the right work and to contribute. All we have to do is ask!

2. Effective questions

In a meeting, you want participants to process information in a useful way that adds value.

Each person in the room is running on a processing question. They are asking themselves a question and continually answering it. By setting that question for them, you can make the meeting much more productive.

Here is how it works: You describe a proposed plan to reorganize the use of contract nurses. As you are speaking, the three questions in people's minds are:

- What is wrong with this proposal?
- Why won't this work?
- Should I support this?

These questions will likely produce negative, highly critical responses. They take the energy out of the room. The response could be defensive. They could generate negative responses.

To create a more productive response, before you speak give the audience the effective questions you want them to address (this is what is meant by framing).

For example:

- What works?

- What do you find exciting?

- In what ways does this contribute to our goals?

- What would you add to make it better?

These are "effective questions" in that they generate positive insights and additions. They are generative; they can't be answered with a yes or no.

3. Active listening

Listening can be a passive activity. As you are listening, you can be distracted, superimposing your own thoughts, drifting away in reverie. Think about the last meeting you were in where you looked around the room and saw people looking at their BlackBerry devices, doodling, gazing out the window, or maybe even nodding off!

Listening is work. In active listening, the listener restates in his or her own language what he or she heard the speaker say and his or her impression of what the speaker said. The speaker can then confirm whether what was heard was what the speaker intended. If it wasn't, the speaker can restate what he or she said. This can continue until the speaker confirms that he or she has been "heard."

Active listening is hard. You have to really listen to what is being said and confirm what is intended to be heard. Active listening gives proof that the listener has understood the speaker.

Another advantage of active listening is that it keeps responsibility for solving the problems with the speaker. If you do not understand what the speaker is intending, it is the speaker's responsibility to explain.

Accountability means doing what you say you are going to do. Often, a lack of accountability is due to miscommunication and unmet expectations. If you are going to hold someone accountable, you need to ensure that this person has heard the expectation and you have heard the commitment to meet the expectation.

In your meetings, frequently ask participants, "What is being said? What are you hearing?"

4. Requests and offers

How many times have you talked about what you needed but not received a response from the room? We are good at describing and explaining, but we are not good at asking.

Requests and offers are one of the most powerful speech acts available to us. This is how you generate commitments. You make requests, you make offers. Most meetings do not end with people leaving in action, because no one made a request and offer. It was assumed that everyone knew what to do.

At some point in the meeting, stop and make requests and offers. You can give each person an opportunity to speak. How do you respond to a request or an offer? You have a choice: Say "yes" or "no." If you say "no," it helps to make a counteroffer. A "no" is often the beginning of a longer conversation.

When you hear a "no," you may need to make a request or an offer. Your request will sound similar to "What would it take for you to be able to say yes?" This reminds me of the last time I bought a car and the dealer asked me, "What would it take for you to buy this car today?" He was asking me to make a commitment.

On our leadership team, we have been practicing using "requests and offers." Using the exact words of *request* and *offer* has provided great cues for action. It helps leaders to think about the commitment they can make or are seeking.

5. Yes/no

When you are talking to someone about accountability, you are often asking the person a simple question: "Are you accountable?" You want to know whether the person is committed to achieving the result under discussion. Too often we hear what we want to, rather than what was said.

Yes/no is about listening for the yes or no. People rarely answer accountability questions with a yes or no. They talk and we mistake their talking for a commitment. We mistake nodding of heads to be a commitment. We mistake "Yes, but . . ." for "Yes."

As leaders and managers, we have to develop an ear for the response. And active listening helps here:

"I am hearing you say that you cannot accept accountability right now because . . . Is that correct?"

As a nursing student, I took a class in therapeutic communication. We learned that we should avoid yes or no questions when establishing a relationship. We were taught to ask leading questions; questions that would get to the why or how of an answer. In accountability, things are different: You are looking for the commitment. This is a yes or no question and we have to hear the "yes" or "no," especially when it is buried under a long explanation.

It is often the "but" or the explanations that can throw you off focus. Consider the following example.

> ## ☑ ACCOUNTABILITY SPOTLIGHT
>
> You are working with a nurse who has a pattern of being 10–15 minutes late most days for her shift. You hold a meeting with her to review what you have observed. She explains that her child is having some adjustment issues in the new school year and she has been driving her child to school, which adds 15 minutes to her morning routine before coming to work. She acknowledges that she understands this is a problem and she feels badly about imposing on her peers. She explains that she has a conference with the teacher tomorrow morning. You meet again the next afternoon, and she says she will be on time each shift. You ask her, "Are you making a commitment that after tomorrow, you will be on time for each shift?" Ideally, she says "yes" and means it.

The scenario might go another way. She might also say something like: "I'll try, but I can't control the traffic. My child might continue to have a problem. You know, I can't control everything. I will do my best." This is a classic "yes, but . . ." answer. If you leave the conversation at this, I can guarantee that there will be no change in the behavior. You have *no* commitment. In an accountability culture, effort is not enough. Accountability is about results; doing what we say we are going to do.

When I am working with a group, I assume that people are rational and logical. So, if I want them to do something, I just need to explain it and they will do it. When I don't get the results I am seeking, I tend to think "Oh, I must not be explaining it well. Let me try it again." It has taken me a long time to realize that what I was hearing as "not understanding me" was often someone's polite way of telling me "no." So, now when I find myself explaining the same thing to someone for the third time, I stop and ask the individual what he or she is hearing me request. If I can validate that the person is hearing me correctly, I ask for the commitment: yes or no.

6. Acknowledgment

We have walked through the steps that can surface commitments and the content and energy that lead to commitments. To get more accountability, we have to acknowledge it when it happens.

Too often we see accountability and almost dismiss it as "someone just doing his or her job." If we succeed in getting someone to make a commitment and, more importantly, keep that commitment, we need to acknowledge and celebrate it.

A version of this practice, published by Doug Krug, is called *DNA*. To get more of what you want, use DNA:

- Define what you want

- Notice it when you get it

- Acknowledge and celebrate it

With the example of the staff nurse who is having difficulty coming to work on time, make sure that on the first day she arrives on time, you acknowledge it. Continue building on her success until there is a pattern, and then a habit. When the nurse has a day where she arrives late, acknowledge that it is not the behavior that is expected and remind her of her past success.

> *"Prior to today you had six days where you were on time. You can be on time. What did you do on those six days to be here on time? What would it take to do those things for your next shift?"*

In essence, you are rewarding/acknowledging the behavior you want to see and the individual is receiving positive reinforcement.

Figure 2.1 is the text from a laminated card I have used with leaders and managers in our organization. There is no magic to the words. We use them as cues to remind us of how we can achieve accountability. I suggest that managers look at the card before they go into a discussion or meeting where they know they are going to try to get a person or a group to be accountable.

FIGURE 2.1: ACCOUNTABILITY POCKET CARD

Make your own pocket card by simply printing this page from the CD-ROM or by copying this page and cutting along the dotted lines. After it is cut out, glue or tape the front of the card to the back of the card and laminate.

Accountability Language

Remember these techniques when practicing or seeking accountability:

Yes/No	Acknowledge
Request and offer	Accountable
Assertions	Calling together
Declarations	Active listening
Stop	Effective questions
Commitment	"And" not "or"
Framing	

Accountability Culture: How We Respond to Attitudes

	Not Accountable	Accountable
No Results	#1. Unacceptable (call it)	#3. Investing for future results
Results	#2. Unacceptable (call it)	#4. Celebration, model

The Power of Accountability Language

As leaders and managers, we are accountable for the productivity of the meetings we are in whether we run the meeting or simply attend it. The six language tools give us a means for fulfilling that accountability.

You can see how powerful they are in that you can use them to turn around very common and frustrating meeting situations that are death to accountability. Specifically, this can produce the following four meeting benefits:

- Create net forward energy up front

- Hold on to the result you want

- Reset meetings that have gone adrift

- Flip negative energy

Create net forward energy

When we are in meetings we are managing the energy. It is almost impossible to get serious accountability established in a negative or low-energy meeting.

Energy comes from the people in the room. We all have been in many low-energy meetings, and even in some toxic meetings. We have been in enough positive-energy meetings to know the difference. We know what we want to see.

A simple and effective way to manage energy is through the concept of "new forward energy" (Krug 1994). The circle in Figure 2.2 represents the meeting.

As people talk, they make statements that add either positive energy (+) or negative energy (-). The negative statements take us back in time. The positive statements take us forward in time. We want the power of the positive statements to outweigh the negative statements.

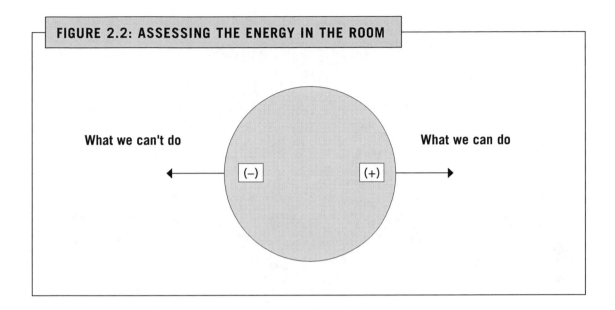

FIGURE 2.2: ASSESSING THE ENERGY IN THE ROOM

What we can't do   (−)   (+)   What we can do

It becomes obvious how to get net positive statements: Learn to make positive statements. Ask others to make positive statements. You have the tools to do this with framing and effective questions.

Have you ever been in a meeting where there is no energy in the room? People are doodling, checking their BlackBerry devices, or making notes about something else. Or maybe you've been in a meeting where one person is talking and the group is expected to sit quietly and listen without responding.

Similarly, have you ever been in a meeting where you suggest a new idea or hear a new idea brought forward by someone else and the response is "That will never work here" or "We tried that a few years ago and it did not work"? These are examples of shutting down positive energy, and such examples cannot be tolerated. You need to call out the "bad story" and not allow it to dampen the positive energy in the conversation.

☑ ACCOUNTABILITY SPOTLIGHT

Bad stories are "called out" at our organization, and here is one example. Several months ago, we held a meeting to plan our implementation of a new predictive hiring model that would allow us to create a pipeline of new hires for our organization so that we could strive to stay ahead of our vacancy curve.

In the meeting, we outlined how we would change our hiring process. An individual in the meeting listened attentively and complimented the group at the end of the meeting for their efforts. His closing comment was "This is a very innovative approach. It's too bad that 'they' probably won't let you do it."

When you hear a bad story such as this, you need to "flip it." When you hear the bad story, you need to understand what you are really hearing. To do this, you must be actively listening. Sometimes what you hear as negative energy or as a bad story is really concern and caring. You need to listen in order to understand, and you need to put yourself in the other person's position. You need to surface the unformed "requests and offers" and seek possible commitment. By actively listening, you restate what you heard the speaker say. Active listening gives proof to the speaker that you understand the speaker's concern. Active listening also keeps the responsibility for solving the problem with the speaker; the person who owns the problem.

In this situation, the response was:

> "I hear that you like our approach and are concerned that we may not be able to implement our idea. How would you suggest we approach the implementation?"

Hold on to the results you want

Let's say you begin a meeting to talk about topic A, a result you want. Suddenly you find yourself on topics B and C, and the meeting ends at X. Later that day you wonder, what happened to the agenda? Using active listening and listening for the yes or no will help you to hold on to the results you want.

☑ ACCOUNTABILITY SPOTLIGHT

A staff nurse who provides excellent patient care is not meeting documentation standards. She consistently leaves work for the next shift, including unfinished documentation. As the nurse manager, you have just had another staff nurse come to you with unfinished admissions paperwork. This staff nurse complains that she does not like to follow this nurse because she always finds charting unfinished or incomplete. She tells you that she has tried to talk to this nurse but the nurse always says how busy she was that shift.

You meet with the nurse to review the specific paperwork that was brought to you. The nurse describes her night to you. She tells you about a difficult patient, a demanding family, and so on. You review her assignment and discuss time management. She tells you she uses time management techniques, but this shift was different. You discuss the pattern you have seen (and discussed with her previously) of unfinished documentation and coaching/mentoring options you have offered (such as the opportunity to observe another nurse who completes documentation, etc.). She acknowledges that you have discussed this with her before and the help she has been offered. She tells you she understands, but she needs to spend the time with her patients.

First of all, count how many "yes, buts . . ." you heard. What is she saying about being accountable? Your response should be: "I appreciate your commitment to caring for our patients. On this unit, I expect that nurses provide quality care. For me, quality care means establishing a trusting relationship with your patients and their loved ones, providing excellent clinical nursing skills, meeting our quality measures, completing documentation as per our standards, and managing your time to do this within your shift. Despite my coaching, you are consistently not meeting our documentation standards. I need to know whether you can commit to meeting our documentation standards. Can you make that commitment?"

She responds: "You know me, I am an excellent nurse here. Of course I want to meet the standards for documentation. So, you just want me to spend less time with my patients?"

Your response: "I expect that you will meet the standards that I have outlined for our unit. If you cannot, perhaps this unit is not the right place for you."

Stop and reset the meeting

Have you ever been in a conversation or a meeting where you are not quite sure why you are there? You don't know what role you are to play or what you are supposed to say. Or the conversation takes a turn down a path other than the one expected. This is a framing problem.

Whenever I am in a meeting, I make sure I know the purpose of the meeting and the role I am to play. Am I going to receive information? Participate in solving a problem? If I don't know "why" I am in the meeting, I ask why.

What I am doing is called *in-the-moment framing*. The original framing didn't happen or it got lost. So, I say, "Stop for a moment." I ask the person who owns the conversation or meeting to reset the conversation by framing. What is the work he or she wants done?

☑ ACCOUNTABILITY SPOTLIGHT

I was recently in a bed meeting with our nurse managers. The day before had been challenging in terms of patient flow. As we were trying to establish the plan for the day, comments about the previous day began to surface. Managers asked questions about what happened, while others explained their actions, and still others tried to ensure that feelings were not hurt. As I sat in the room, I could feel the emotions start to incite. Comments vacillated from accusatory to apologetic to defensive. I stood up and declared, "Stop! What are we doing? There is no blaming or punishment. Is there anything from yesterday that you would do differently?" This question allowed the group to "reset" and answer questions without affixing blame.

In another meeting, I had invited managers from another department to meet with nurse managers for us to strategize on a plan for a program implementation. We proceeded through the agenda, and once during the meeting I felt like we had lost track of the agenda, so I declared, "Stop, can we just check where we are? Where are we in the agenda? Is everyone clear on where we are?" By stopping the conversation, I gave people the opportunity to ask questions without feeling like they were out of place.

Flip negative energy in the room

Here is a situation you can encounter every day. The conversation has turned negative. The room is full of bad stories about others. It contains a lot of "we can't, they won't" neqativity.

The good news is that there is energy in the room! Now you have the tools to flip the negative energy and make it positive. With active listening, requests and offers, and acknowledgment, you have enough to get the source of the negativity into positive action. Take a look at Figure 2.3.

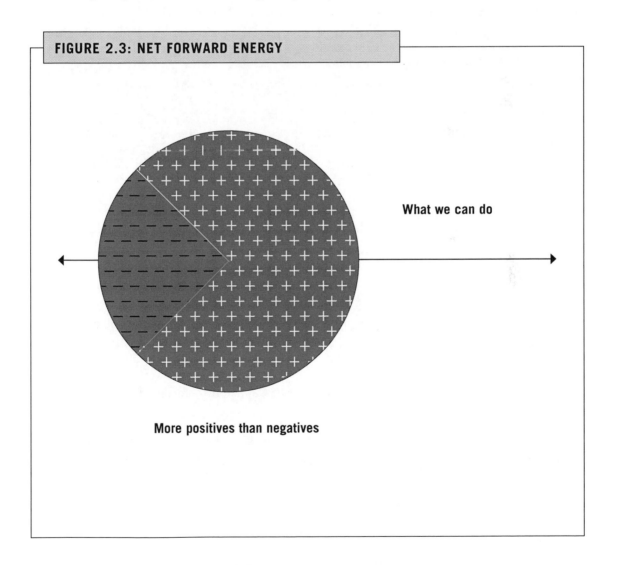

FIGURE 2.3: NET FORWARD ENERGY

What we can do

More positives than negatives

☑ ACCOUNTABILITY SPOTLIGHT

Recently I was meeting with our home health managers. They were voicing concern over their progress in improving their performance in one area. The conversation was negative. And as each person spoke, the energy in the room became even more negative.

I stopped the meeting and worked to flip the negative energy. I told them that I heard their concern about the progress. I also told them I heard them making an offer. I asked whether they were offering to create a new approach to their work; a new campaign that would require a strong partnership with other departments. I suggested they could start meeting weekly on these issues. Within a few moments, each manager was making suggestions about who should be at the weekly meetings, the topics to be discussed, and the plans to be made.

Develop a New Habit and Track Your Progress

Want to have some fun with this? Here is a simple exercise that I know you will find fascinating. The exercise involves collecting data on the meetings you are in.

Keep a log for the next week. In that log, rate the productivity of every meeting you are in on a scale of 1 to 5, with 1 meaning low productivity and 5 meaning high productivity. Count productivity as the number of commitments made in the meeting to produce a result. Keep track of how many people attended, how long the meeting was, and how many people left in action.

At the end of the week, add the number of meetings and get the average score. Look for outliers for insight. What was the best meeting and what made it best? What was the least productive, and what made it so?

With this as your baseline, begin to practice using the tools presented in this chapter. For a few subsequent weeks keep the log and see whether you can improve the ratings.

I know you can!

REFERENCES

Oakley, E., and D. Krug. 1994. *Enlightened Leadership: Getting to the Heart of Change.* New York: Simon and Schuster.

PERSONAL ACCOUNTABILITY

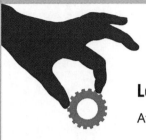

Learning Objectives

After reading this chapter, the participant will be able to:

- Identify your personal level of accountability

- Examine your personal communication style

- Describe how to use accountability language and behavior

Identifying Your Personal Level of Accountability

Accountability is about making and keeping commitments, and it starts with you. To demonstrate that you are accountable you need to ask yourself what it will take for you to make a commitment.

Start with yourself

Do you practice accountability? Do you do what you say you will do? Do others believe they can count on you?

It is unrealistic to expect accountability of others if you don't expect it of yourself. Accountability exists in all facets of your life, and in every relationship. Practicing accountability will affect all the relationships in your life. It is about expectations and commitments. If you do not understand what is expected of you, you will not be successful in meeting commitments, even though you may work very hard to be accountable. It starts with clearly understanding what the other person is expecting.

Have you ever been in a situation where you did what you thought was expected and then found out that something else was expected? For example, your spouse asks you to pick up bread on your way home. You stop and buy a loaf of white bread. You bring it home to your spouse, who tells you that he or she actually wanted whole wheat bread and won't eat white bread. This is a very simple example, but it demonstrates the point. If you don't understand what is expected, you will never be able to keep commitments.

So, let's assess your ability to be accountable. When you say you are going to do something, do you mean it? Do you commit to things that are realistic? Do you ensure that you understand what is expected of you? If you realize that you cannot keep a commitment, do you communicate this in a timely manner? Do you ask for help when making commitments and working on them?

I have worked with many people who tell me they are accountable for something. Yet time and again, they do not meet expectations or deliver on commitments they have made. Their intentions are good, but their performance is not acceptable. Compounding the situation, their explanation for not meeting the expectation is usually filled with excuses and blame—neither of which has a place in an accountability culture.

Accountability often means you have to engage others to help you keep your commitments. Some people find this to be the most challenging part of accountability—depending on others. Many times, we need the help of others for us to be accountable.

Identify sore spots

It is important to understand what prevents you from meeting expectations, making a commitment, and keeping a commitment. You need to understand your sore spots: the situations, individuals, or groups that threaten your ability to be accountable.

When someone in authority asks you to do something, do you say "yes" regardless of whether you mean it because of the position of the person who is asking you?

Is there an individual who you have a hard time saying "no" to, such as a friend or sibling? You don't want to let this person down, so you say "yes," but you may not be willing or able to do what this person is requesting.

Is there a team whose help you need, so you say "yes" to their request of you so that they will say "yes" when you have to make a request of them?

When you are not clear on what is expected of you, ask questions—make requests—until you understand what is expected, how it will be measured, and the time expectation for its completion.

Tell Your Accountability Story

When you are accountable, don't be afraid to tell your accountability story.

I wear a button that says, "Ask me what I am accountable for." I am most amazed when I meet visitors on the hospital elevator who will indeed ask me, "What are you accountable for?" I respond, "I am accountable for all of the nursing care that is provided in this building."

I know my accountability story is true when families or visitors tell me about their patient care experience in our hospital. Whether positive or negative, they find me and hold me accountable for the care that was received. I don't provide any of the care. Yet I have to know that we provide excellent care. I know that from what I observe, what nurses tell me, and the many measures we have in place to demonstrate excellent patient care.

What are you accountable for? Don't be afraid to tell others. A public declaration of what you are accountable for can help support your efforts and results.

Think about when a friend starts a diet. When your friend tells you he or she has started dieting, what is your response? Do you find yourself watching what your friend eats? Maybe even reminding your friend if you see him or her eating a cookie? A public declaration can help you to engage others in your work.

Accountability allows you to meet expectations because you ensure that you understand what is expected, how the expectation will be measured, and the time when it is to be delivered.

It comes down to the how to "be" that we discussed in previous chapters. How do you need to "be"? Are you actively listening? Are you making requests and offers?

Your Communication Style

How effectively do you communicate? Your accountability language can help you be an effective communicator. It will help you to clearly communicate your expectations.

In bad times

When you are faced with challenges, it is easy to fall into the trap of blame and excuses. In an accountability culture, there is no blame or punishment. These create negative energy and cause you to lose focus on the goal. When you are in a difficult situation and are tempted to break into a "bad story," remember that accountability is about clear expectations and making and keeping commitments. When commitments are not met, you need to understand what happened. What went well? The answer to this question is meant to create positive energy to generate more new ideas.

Your language and behavior

Being accountable does not mean you can always do what is being requested. You may not be able to say "yes" to a request. The important part of accountability is that you commit to something. It is your job to make a commitment that you understand and can keep. If you cannot, you need to adjust the commitment to what you can achieve. Remember, use your accountability language to help you make and keep commitments (Figure 3.1).

FIGURE 3.1: ACCOUNTABILITY LANGUAGE

- Declaration
- Framing
- Acknowledge
- Accountable
- Say "yes"
- Calling together
- Request and offer
- Active listening
- Effective questions
- Assertions
- "And" not "or"

How you speak will let others know that you understand what is expected.

Nonverbal communication

Watch your nonverbal communication, too. Sometimes what you don't say reveals much more about your accountability. Take, for instance, a meeting you are in where everyone seems to be committing to doing something: heads are nodding, people are smiling, and everyone seems to be engaged. In reality, the people walking out of the room are saying to themselves, "I have no idea what they were talking about. I just said 'yes' so that we could get out of there." Pay attention to whether you are behaving in the same way.

Personal Accountability Situations

When you are not being accountable, you are not making commitments and/or not keeping the commitments you have made. There can be many legitimate reasons for not being accountable. Sometimes you may not be able to be accountable. In other situations, not being accountable looks like poor performance.

Let's say you are the nursing supervisor who oversees patient placement or flow. You work with staff nurses on all units to place patients in the appropriate beds. One evening, the emergency department is particularly busy with admissions. As you are placing patients, you receive resistance from several units who say they cannot accept admissions due to low staffing.

As a patient placement supervisor, you can do everything right with the placement process, but your role does not include staffing; you are responsible for the patient placement process, but you are not accountable for staffing and making sure every unit has sufficient staff members to accept all admissions. For you to be successful with patient placement, you will need to engage nurse managers, as they are accountable for staffing. For the patient placement to work the nursing supervisor must follow the placement process *and* the nurse managers must ensure that staffing is adequate and that they hold their staff accountable to accept admissions.

In another situation, a lack of accountability can be very obvious. Let's say you make a commitment to do something that you are not sure you can do. You don't raise your concern when making the commitment, either because you think you might be able to make the commitment or because you are not comfortable telling the person who is asking for the commitment that you cannot do what is requested. With all good intentions, you are not able to keep the commitment.

This is another example where your accountability language is critical.

When someone asks you to make a commitment, he or she is making a request. You respond with a "yes" or a "no." You can also respond with an offer—an offer to be accountable with some changes to the initial request. You can assert what you will do and make a commitment to what you know you can achieve or know you have the likelihood to achieve.

Another difficult situation is when you are asked to make a commitment and you are uncomfortable saying "no" to the request. For example, you are in a bed meeting on a day when the census is very high and inpatient admissions are being held in the emergency department. You have several empty beds on your unit, but the patients in the emergency department are not the patient population you usually have on your unit or you do not have enough staff members for the empty beds. The vice president of nursing asks you to take five of the inpatient admissions from the emergency department to your empty beds. You know that saying "no" is not acceptable, so you say "yes" but you have no idea how you will be able to care for the patients. After leaving the meeting, you talk to the patient placement coordinator and tell her that you will not be able to accept the emergency department admissions. A short time later, the vice president of nursing calls you and asks why the patients were not moved from the emergency room to your empty rooms.

A person who is accountable would handle that situation by responding to the vice president's initial request during the bed meeting with an offer:

> *"I have five empty beds. All of the patients in the emergency room need telemetry, and my unit does not do telemetry. Instead of taking the patients from the emergency room, I will work with the patient flow coordinator to see whether there are five patients in the 'house' who do not need telemetry and could be transferred to my unit. This will free up the beds that the emergency room needs. We should be able to complete this in the next two to three hours. Will that be acceptable?"*

It is important to know when a request is being made and someone is asking you to be accountable. Before making a commitment, you need to understand the request that is being made and the commitment that is being sought. Remember, you need to understand the expectations: the results that are expected and the time by which they are expected to be achieved. If you are not sure of the expectations, how they will be measured, or when they are to be delivered, you need to make additional requests before you make a commitment.

Accountability starts with you. It is about doing what you will say you will do and getting others to make commitment to you. Now that you understand the role you plan in accountability, let's apply these ideas, tools and techniques with others.

CHAPTER 4

HOLDING STAFF MEMBERS ACCOUNTABLE

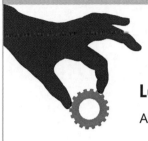

Learning Objectives

After reading this chapter, the participant will be able to:

- Discuss how managers can set accountability expectations

- Describe how to hold staff accountable in a variety of work settings and situations

Defining Accountability and Expectations for Your Staff

Nurse managers are in one of the most difficult roles in any organization: They must manage nursing units while supervising, leading, and mentoring the nursing staff.

To be effective managers and to promote the organization's goals of patient safety, patient satisfaction, and high-quality care, nurse managers rely on staff nurses to provide excellent patient care and to follow the organization's policies and procedures. Nurse managers want staff nurses who are skilled clinicians and are driven to provide excellent care using critical thinking skills. Nurse managers want staff nurses who are committed to providing excellent patient care through interdisciplinary practice, focusing on best practices and evidence-based practice. Nurse managers want staff nurses who value evidence-based practice and understand how to seek and utilize it.

Every other week I welcome new nurses to our hospital. I share my first "cardinal rule" with them: When you leave this orientation classroom and come to your unit, I don't want you to do anything unless you understand:

- What you are doing

- Why you are doing it

- The effect it has on the world around you

I explain that for those who hold a license, like I do, this is called "safe practice" and is a requirement for how we practice at our hospital.

Lack of accountability

Gather any group of nurse managers together, and one of the complaints heard most often concerns the lack of accountability among the staff. The most common question I hear from nurse managers is, "How can I get the staff to be accountable?"

As nurse managers, we become frustrated when accountability does not occur and people do not do what we expect them to do. How many times have you wondered why your staff's performance does not meet your expectations?

You can answer this question and find ways to improve staff accountability by examining the reasons why staff nurses fail to be accountable. Many times, it is because the request was not understood, meaning the nurses will not meet the expectations because they do not understand what those expectations are. Other times, it is because staff nurses do not accept the expectation and do not make the commitment to meet the expectation.

Nurse managers spend a great deal of time and energy communicating and recommunicating their intent, which is time well spent if the nurses simply do not understand the intent on first delivery. But if you fail to gain any assurance that your staff nurses are making real commitments, you are not spending your time wisely.

Engaging in Effective Conversations

The key to accountability is clearly communicated expectations. We need to be careful not to "assume" that staff nurses know what is expected of them. We need to set clear expectations and communicate them, including the consequences of not meeting the expectations.

I cannot stress this point enough. A nurse manager needs to clearly tell staff nurses what they are accountable for, gain their commitment to meet the expectation, and then hold them to that accountability. Having staff nurses repeat the expectation back to you in their own words is an effective tool to ensure that they understand what is expected of them and what they are committing to achieve. A breakdown in any step will result in a lack of accountability.

☑ ACCOUNTABILITY SPOTLIGHT

Let's think of a new nurse on a unit. Medication reconciliation is an area of focus for this unit. The nurse is informed of this focus and the nurse manager tells him that the Core Measures nurse reviews all discharged charts to ensure that medication reconciliation is completed. The nurse is oriented to the medication reconciliation documentation and process. Several weeks later, the nurse manager talks to this nurse to report that his medication reconciliation documentation is incomplete. The nurse explains that he performs the medication reconciliation process as instructed, as best he can, knowing that his work is checked by the Core Measures nurse. The nurse says, "Sometimes I am very busy with the discharge teaching, so I don't always get to document all of the discharge meds. I know the Core Measures nurse will be reviewing the chart, so she will catch this and finish it for me."

The nurse manager may be disappointed with this response, but she needs to ask herself: Did I clearly convey the expectation that the staff nurse needed to complete all of the medication reconciliation documentation himself and not rely on the Core Measures nurse to do or check his work?

Getting staff nurses to be consistently accountable is a nurse manager's challenge. Paying attention to the distinction between *accountability* and *responsibility* will help nurse managers determine what is happening and set commitments that can be kept. Remember the difference between responsibility and accountability:

- **Responsibility:** I have authority over things and they will respond to me

- **Accountability:** I am committed to others to deliver and account for results by a given date

Nurse managers can engage nurses in at least three different accountability conversations, each intended to generate commitments on performance. To demonstrate this, let's examine the example of hourly rounding.

A unit has adopted the process of hourly rounding as a method to improve patient satisfaction. Nurses are expected to round each hour on their patients, and to use a script that involves checking on the three Ps: pain, position, and potty.

Three levels of conversation occur:

- **Level 1:** Nurses are asked to be professionally responsible for the care they deliver. In this example, it is rounding with their patients every hour. The concept of accountability here is soft, since it becomes "be accountable for doing what you are responsible for doing." There is no outcome beyond the activity.

- **Level 2:** Nurses are asked to be accountable for the outcome of their care, such as patient satisfaction. Nurses are accountable and responsible. Nurses have control over their own practice and they can adjust that practice to achieve the outcome for which they are accountable.

- **Level 3:** Nurses are asked to be accountable for the unit's outcomes—in this case, patient satisfaction scores for the care given. This involves unit activities beyond individual nurses' responsibilities. Nurses are accountable but not responsible. To be effective, they will have to collaborate with fellow nurses who collectively have the responsibility to deliver the outcome. It's the nursing team that is accountable and responsible for unit performance. The individual nurses share the accountability.

Each of these conversations addresses responsibility and accountability. When a staff nurse is doing his or her job, the staff nurse is responsible for doing what his or her job description defines. This is the case in Level 1. As you move into the scenarios described in Levels 2 and 3, the nurse must influence other nurses' practices. As the nurse talks to a coworker about a conversation she observed between a staff nurse and a patient and suggests how the observed nurse might respond differently to achieve higher patient satisfaction, the nurse is trying to influence the behavior of another nurse, yet she is not the nurse's supervisor.

You may begin to see why conversations about accountability can be confusing and can fail to pin down the desired commitments. As managers move from Level 1 to 2 to 3, they need a framework to make distinctions so that they are clear about their expectations. Nurse managers need a game plan where they translate their intentions (expectations) into these three conversations.

COMMITMENT TIP

To secure commitment from a staff member:

- Express clear intent

- Communicate expectations

- Verify that you were heard

- Hear and verify the response

To get a staff member to deliver on commitments:

- Monitor performance

- Create pacing events that acknowledge delivery on commitments

- Fine-tune commitments and energize them through ongoing accountability conversations

- Clean up failure to deliver on commitments

Conversations that hold nurses accountable

When a new nurse starts on the unit, the nurse manager has an accountability conversation with the nurse. As part of the orientation process, the manager tells the new nurse that she expects nurses to do hourly rounding with all patients. The nurse manager describes the studies showing that customer service scores are high—greater than the 85th percentile—when organizations use this practice. The manager explains that it is each nurse's responsibility to conduct hourly rounding with his or her patients and that the unit uses a script that engages patients and a checklist of activities to conduct with patients. The unit also regularly holds training demonstrations within the unit to sharpen everyone's skills.

Now the nurse manager must determine whether the new nurse understands the process and the expectations, so she asks the staff nurse what he hears. The manager expects the new nurse to be able to express the policy in his own words. The nurse manager also asks the nurse what he finds exciting or interesting about the policy and the nurse manager expects him to be intrigued by the results it can deliver. In this unit, the manager expects nurses to see hourly rounding as part of their professional practice.

As the nurse talks about the practice, the manager is looking for him to accept responsibility for rounding. Does the nurse accept responsibility? The manager must ask for a commitment to hourly rounding. At this point, the manager is listening for the nurse to say "yes." But in many situations, you will not hear a simple "yes" or "no." Instead, you will hear nurses talk a lot about the practice.

Staff nurse:

> *"I always see my patients frequently. Of course, sometimes we get busy. We do have a lot of paperwork. My patients have always expressed satisfaction with my service. What I love about nursing is taking care of patients."*

Does the manager have a commitment? Not yet. The manager needs to determine whether she is hearing a "no," or whether the nurse is requesting help so that he can say "yes."

Nurse manager:

> *"I hear you saying that you may need help with managing your paperwork so that you can have the time to round each hour. Are you committing to do the hourly rounding and do you need help with the paperwork?"*

Staff nurse:

> *"It's more than the paperwork that takes up our time. Yes, I will do the hourly rounding to the best of my ability."*

Does the manager have a commitment? No. The manager has a "yes, but . . ." response, and the "but" negates the "yes." The phrase "to the best of my ability" makes the statement ambiguous, and therefore negates the "yes."

Nurse manager:

> *"Let me restate the policy. Every nurse does hourly rounding with his or her patients. Are you able to make a commitment to do that?"*

If the staff nurse responds with a lengthy explanation, the nurse manager simply asks, "Is that a 'yes'?" In the end, it is imperative that the manager hears a "yes" or a "no."

If the nurse responds "no," the manager must have a different conversation with the nurse. The manager must determine whether this unit is the best fit for the nurse in the organization. By responding "no," the nurse is choosing not to work on this unit. The manager may offer the nurse the chance to look for other opportunities in the organization where he may find a better fit regarding his professional practice.

If the nurse responds "yes," the manager can be confident that she has received a verbal commitment. This is not the end of the process—the manager must now hold the nurse accountable for the commitment by monitoring whether he keeps the commitment.

Continuing with the rounding example, let's say several weeks have passed and the nurse manager has noticed that the staff nurse is not always rounding every hour. The nurse manager's first response is to remind the staff nurse of the expectation and to coach him on how to conduct hourly rounding and meet his commitment.

If times goes by and the staff nurse continues to not meet the expectation, the manager has to reengage him in the accountability conversation.

Staff nurse:

> *"It's not fair to say I have not been meeting my commitment to round with my patients. I have been rounding whenever I can. But during the last four hours of my shift, there are too many things to do. Sometimes I cannot get to it, but with good reason."*

Nurse manager:

> *"I hear that you are committed to rounding and that you need help with your workload and time management at the end of the shift. Are you requesting help with your time management? I can have one of our senior nurses work with you. What I need from you is assurance that you are responsible for the hourly rounding."*

The nurse has a choice. He can recommit to the practice and accept the help he needs to perform to expectations. Or he can choose to leave the unit and work in a situation that better fits his style. This conversation does not involve blame or punishment. It is simply not accepting nonperformance.

Intolerance of nonperformance

Nurse managers often see pockets of nonperformance among their staff members, and many times it seems easy to forgive, accept, or overlook these instances since those nurses do many others things well. But nurse managers need to examine their level of tolerance, as tolerating a lack of accountability sends a powerful message to your other staff members who are being accountable.

> *"She is a very good nurse, but she doesn't document well. She especially has trouble with discharge. But she tries. No one is perfect."*

This is unacceptable. As nurse managers, we must hold all nurses to the same level of accountability. We can do this by training nurses in the process or procedure or whatever it is that we want them to do, and then ask them to commit to being accountable for a specific practice.

Nurse managers cannot accept nonperformance. In the example concerning documentation, the nurse manager must engage the nurse in conversation and make a request: Will you commit to our documentation policy?

Then listen for the answer:

Yes	The nurse commits.
Yes, and . . .	The nurse commits and requests assistance.
No	The nurse chooses not to commit.
Yes, but . . .	The nurse says "yes" but negates it with qualifiers.

In the case of "yes, but . . ." the conversation must continue until the ambiguity is resolved.

Facilitating Effective Staff Meetings

Nurse managers have many opportunities to expect accountability from their staff members, both during one-on-one interactions and in group settings. An area where nurse managers should expect accountability, but where they frequently complain they see none, is during staff meetings.

Nurse managers can promote accountability during meetings by setting expectations and facilitating the meeting so that staff nurses know how to behave.

When starting a staff meeting, the manager must "set the stage" for how he or she wants the staff to "be" in the meeting. The manager should tell the staff whether the meeting will involve them receiving information, whether they will be asked to give feedback, whether they will be asked to make a decision, and so on. Every meeting will be more effective if those in the meeting know what is expected of them.

One way to prepare staff members for a meeting is to set an agenda ahead of time. Having an agenda that is available prior to the meeting can set the stage for what is expected and alerts staff members to how they need to "be" in the meeting (see Figure 4.1).

FIGURE 4.1: HOW TO "BE" IN A MEETING

Leading a Meeting

When you are leading a meeting, you need to "frame" the meeting at the beginning so that your attendees understand how they need to "be" in that meeting.

Tell attendees:

- Role you want them to play
    - Leader
    - Manager
    - Staff
- Purpose of the meeting
- Anticipated work to be done
- Anticipated outcome of the meeting
- Agenda of the meeting
    - What is the expectation
- How they should handle requests and offers

Attending a Meeting

When you are attending a meeting, prepare for how you should "be" in the meeting.

Questions you may ask prior to the meeting—or early in the meeting—include:

- What role do I play in the meeting?
- What work will be done?
    - Information sharing/update
    - Problem solving
    - Strategic thinking
- What is the anticipated outcome of the meeting?

In a meeting, staff members need to understand what is expected of them. Are they there to be reported to? Hear, understand, and assimilate information? Provide feedback? Another important part of an effective meeting is the commitment and follow-up. If staff members are to be involved in the staff meeting and unit performance, they need to be asked what they are committing to and the manager needs to know (and communicate!) what the follow-up to the commitment will be.

Have you ever been in a meeting where everyone seemed engaged? Heads are nodding, and suggestions and ideas are flowing. Several months later you are in another meeting to discuss the same problem as before. You are convinced that the issue was resolved and you ask what happened after the last meeting. Although it may have appeared that everyone was committed, no one person had assumed accountability for the meeting and no one person had driven everyone on the unit to achieve the results.

> **☑ ACCOUNTABILITY SPOTLIGHT**
>
> For example, during the weekly staff meeting the nurse manager introduces a new initiative to cut back on overtime. The manager tells everyone that reports show that overtime has increased significantly on the unit during the previous two months. Some of the attendees reveal displeasure, and others a lack of interest.
>
> As the attendees talk, the following comments are heard:
>
> - "This will hurt quality"
>
> - "All the administration worries about is money"
>
> Others begin to talk about why the overtime is happening:
>
> - "Our patients are sicker."
>
> - "We have been short-staffed."
>
> - "The other policy has been to reduce travelers. We have used overtime to meet need when travelers left."
>
> Now there is a lot of negative energy in the room and the nurse manager cannot receive commitments from the staff under these conditions. When the energy is negative, you cannot have an effective conversation about accountability.
>
> The manager must turn the negative energy around.

Flipping negative energy

Let's examine a different example to see how someone can turn negative energy around. A nursing director is in a staff meeting with the management team of a home health and hospice unit in a large hospital. They are discussing whether to agree to a policy where they will accept new patients who are being discharged from the hospital. To do so, they will need to increase staff levels so that they can provide services to these patients.

The idea quickly generates complaints, and many are worried that the growth and capability to provide care will be constrained by the limited availability of physical therapists. One of the clinical managers expresses frustration and lays blame:

> *"It is very hard to find physical therapists. There aren't very many PTs out there. I just don't see how we will be able to do this."*

This statement triggers others to share bad stories about past recruiting and hiring experiences. The conversation is going toxic and the energy in the room is negative. Immediately the director moves to flip the negative energy.

Director:

> *"I hear you are frustrated. I hear a request that we enter into a new partnership with HR. You would like to investigate some creative recruitment ideas with them."*

There is silence in the room for a moment. The director turns to the original speaker:

> *"Are you offering to lead the effort to establish a new relationship with HR?"*

The original speaker does not respond immediately. The other participants begin to brainstorm ways to set up this new partnership and begin to throw out innovative recruiting and hiring initiatives. As comfort with this new idea grows, commitments are made to consider new approaches.

The director has successfully flipped negative energy by using three tools:

- Active listening: "I hear you are frustrated . . ."

- Hearing the request below the surface: "And I hear a request that . . ."

- Surfacing the possible offer: "Are you offering to lead . . .?"

By turning the gripe session into an accountability conversation, the director flipped negative energy into positive energy, and the crucial part was doing so in the moment. Sometimes negative energy can be an asset. It means we have touched something people care about and with which they have an emotional connection. We have their attention; they are engaged. Rather than shut down the negativity, or let it run amok, turn it into something productive by flipping it into a positive track.

Professional Staff Development

As managers, we are responsible for the professional development of our staff members. We must support staff members to achieve results and to sustain those results, and this depends on accountability. Staff members need to understand what is expected of them. When we provide them with expectations that are defined, measurable, and time-limited, they have choices. They can choose to meet the expectations. If they need assistance or support to meet the expectations, they can make "requests" or "offers" that will allow them to achieve the expected results.

For a new graduate nurse, professional development starts during orientation. Nurse managers and preceptors must invest in developing critical thinking skills in the new nurse. These develop through coaching the new nurse in patient care situations. The new nurse is continually expected to understand what he or she is doing, why he or she is doing it, and the effect his or her intervention is having on the patient as well as on the world around the patient. The nurse is expected to use the interdisciplinary team to assist in achieving the expected outcomes for the patient. As clear expectations are identified and communicated, and performance is monitored to achieve the expectations, the new nurse is being held accountable.

As a nurse develops proficiency and accountability in a staff role, we continue to communicate expectations for expanded roles such as charge nurse, unit educator, and perhaps eventually, nurse manager. If additional education is an option, we communicate what will be expected and support this continued professional development.

Throughout professional development, clearly communicated expectations and monitoring of the performance of these expectations are necessary. Holding someone accountable is not a single event. Accountability is important in sustaining results. Our staff nurses need to understand that sustaining results is as important as, and often more difficult than, achieving results. As you coach and support someone by communicating clear expectations and holding him or her accountable to achieve the clear expectations, you need to be prepared to do this again and again. A danger in holding someone accountable is that you must sustain the expectations and not waver.

☑ ACCOUNTABILITY SPOTLIGHT

Take, for example, the nurse who has improved her documentation on discharge instructions for a congestive heart failure (CHF) patient. As the nurse meets the expectations, you utilize DNA. You have (D) defined what you want (discharge instruction components are clearly documented on discharge). When the nurse does this you (N) notice the success of meeting this expectation. The nurse does this on several CHF patients, so you continue to (A) acknowledge the behavior.

A couple of weeks later, you notice that one of her CHF discharge charts does not have discharge instructions documented. You tell yourself, "Oh, they were very busy last night; she has done so well," and decide not to address the incident. You have just allowed/enabled a lack of accountability and should expect to see the results that you have tolerated continue: no discharge instructions documented on every CHF patient from now on. You also have to be consistent: What is a clear expectation today has to be the same expectation tomorrow. Holding staff nurses accountable is hard work and takes a commitment on the part of the manager.

The DNA tool can be useful. As you define what you expect and notice it when it is achieved, you provide positive reinforcement to your staff for the behavior/results you want to see and you acknowledge and celebrate with them. However, your greatest challenge will be sustaining the results. This requires a commitment on the part of the manager to *always* clearly communicate expectations *and* hold people to the expectations regardless of anything else going on.

Promoting Intolerance

As managers, we also need to develop an intolerance to lack of accountability. We cannot excuse the lack of accountability we may see. We may encounter lack of accountability in our staff, peers, supervisors, physicians, and senior leadership. I often hear managers say, "I hold my staff accountable, but other managers don't." When I ask about holding everyone accountable, I hear, "Oh, I can only control my staff."

As you work to create a culture of accountability, everyone needs to be in the game. In my organization, we are working to improve our service culture. One behavior we have addressed concerns greeting people we encounter in the hallway with a simple "Hello," "Good morning," and so forth. In a follow-up leadership meeting, we discussed this expectation and communicated challenges. One attendee said, "I say hello to everyone I see in the hallway and some people just don't even respond." When asked what he does about that behavior, he did not respond. After further discussion, attendees agreed that whenever a leader greeted a staff member and did not receive a response, the leader would stop and address the behavior with comments such as "Hey there, I just said good morning and you did not respond. Is everything okay?" Or "Hello, good morning. You must have a number of things on your mind. I just said hello to you and you did not answer me. Are you okay?" After several weeks, leaders reported that anyone they had addressed was now saying hello each time they encountered him or her in the hallway.

We also need to be intolerant of poor meetings and poor communication. If expectations need to be communicated in clear, definable, measurable, and time-limited terms to generate accountability, we must be intolerant of expectations that are not communicated in this way. Accountability is hard work. Accountability means making and keeping commitments. Holding people accountable is about being committed to expecting people to keep their commitments. This takes time, so time spent in meetings where we do not hold people accountable is not time well spent, and we need to create the environment where this is not tolerable.

We've all been in a meeting in which we are discussing the same problem we thought we had resolved in a meeting 10 months before. As the meeting churns on, a new plan is developed and everyone in the room seems to agree to it. What is different this time? If nothing is different, you can expect the same results: no change. The problem is that although there is a plan, no one was identified as accountable, or if someone was identified as accountable, that person did not keep his or her commitment and the results were the same: no change. Rather than spending or wasting time on another plan, this behavior needs to be "called" in the meeting. Accountability means that someone is accountable to produce a desired, measurable result by a specific date. Accountability is not about effort—in other words, "I did my best." Accountability is about the committed results.

Now, in an accountability culture, sometimes a commitment cannot be kept. For example, say that a plan is agreed to and someone is identified as accountable. However, something in the plan does not work as planned or something unexpected happens during the plan. In that situation, the accountable individual needs to come back to the group, explain the problem, and provide a new plan of what results can be achieved and by when. For those of you who are familiar with performance improvement methodologies, this is time to use the plan, do, check, act (PDCA) strategy. You design a plan, implement or do something, and then check the results. If you are not achieving the desired results, you act—perhaps by going back to the plan and revising the "do" to achieve the desired, measurable results by the committed time.

In a meeting, it is also critical that you understand the role you are being asked to play. Are you there to receive information? Are you there to provide direction or input? Or are you there as a team member or as a supervisor? For example, our CEO has a weekly meeting with the executive team. A portion of his meeting is clearly devoted to providing updates. During this time in the meeting, my role is clear: I am listening for information that I need to know to do my job. Sometimes I am invited to a meeting with a group who is resolving a problem. I need to know whether I am there in my role as vice president; this usually means they want me to tell some-one what to do (not as much fun) or they are requesting my expertise to work with them to address the solution (much more fun for me). Take a look at Figure 4.2 for a meeting redesign tool, and Figure 4.3 for a commitment log.

As a manager and leader, we are always needing staff to do something. The accountability tools and techniques discussed in this chapter will help you to get your staff to do what you need. They will make and most importantly keep commitments.

In my opinion, the role of the nurse manager is the hardest role in the hospital. I like to equate it with the cream inside an Oreo cookie. One chocolate wafer is your staff pushing on you to meet their needs. The other wafer is made up of the people like me, the nurse leader or executive, who hold you accountable for the operation and outcomes of your unit. In this chapter, I have offered techniques and tools that I hope will help you preserve and safeguard the cream!

FIGURE 4.2: MEETING REDESIGN TOOL

One of our hospitalwide shared governance councils is the Nursing Leadership Council (NLC). The council meets monthly and membership is comprised of all nursing directors, managers, and the vice president of nursing. Each member has one vote. It is chaired by a nurse manager and the chair has a one-year term.

Recently, one of our nursing leadership retreats examined how to make nurse leaders' time more valuable and examined meetings that did not bring value. NLC was identified as a meeting that did not bring value to the nursing leaders. This monthly, two-hour meeting was described as "flat," "boring," and "unproductive."

So we set out to revise the meeting, and several months later, leaders describe the meeting as "interesting" and say they "don't want to miss it." Here's how we did it.

Redesign of NLC

Nonnursing leadership always viewed the NLC as the best way to communicate information to all nursing leadership. People would request to present at NLC and they would be added to the agenda. All too often, they would present information that nursing already knew about, or they would exceed their time on the agenda, or provide information that nursing leadership did not understand, or request support from nursing without presenting adequate details. And they never brought enough handouts.

New Design

The council meeting is now run in a completely different way. Anyone who wants to be on the NLC agenda must make a request to the NLC leader. The leader meets with anyone on the agenda prior to the meeting to review what is to be presented, including format and time needed. The NLC leader also reviews presentation slides and handouts, if used.

Each presenter is told how much time they will have and requested to have a sufficient number of handouts available at the beginning of the meeting so they can be distributed to all attendees. The NLC leader creates and distributes the agenda to NLC members.

At the meeting, the NLC leader selects two cohosts for each presentation (cohosts are NLC members). That day's speaker is asked to direct his or her presentation to the cohosts. While all members hear the presentation, the cohosts have the task of hearing the presentation on behalf of all in attendance. After the presentation, the cohosts restate what they heard in the presentation. If the presenter has made any requests of the NLC, the cohosts restate the request and then lead the NLC in discussion so that they may respond to the request.

It is the cohosts who respond to the presenter. If NLC has requests or offers to make to the presenter, the cohosts make those requests or offers on behalf of the NLC.

FIGURE 4.3: COMMITMENT LOG

We have recently begun using a commitment log in many meetings. The commitment log is a form completed by each manager where they identify what they have committed to in the meeting.

For example, at a recent meeting we were reviewing our performance in medication reconciliation and unit-based shared governance participation. We identified both areas as opportunities for improvement. We reviewed practices on units with better performance than others and, as a group, we committed to use the identified best practices.

Each manager was asked to complete the commitment log to publicly record what they were committing to do on their unit. The commitment log was submitted to the vice president of nursing and each manager kept a copy of his or her commitments.

We have adapted the commitment log for future meetings and here is an example of the commitment log relating to medication reconciliation.

Nursing Leadership Retreat Commitment Log

Manager: _____

Unit: _____ Date: _____

Medication reconciliation

Stand: I am committing to improve my unit's performance in medication reconciliation to
_____ by _____.
   (% compliance)   (date)

I am committed to sharing best practices with other nurse managers.

Method: The way I will accomplish this is by adopting the best practices of 5 South (best practice unit) including:

_____

_____

_____

FIGURE 4.3: COMMITMENT LOG (CONT.)

Accountability: I will measure my unit's performance each week by:

_____

_____

_____

Unit-based shared governance participation

Stand: I am committing to improve participation in my unit's shared governance council to

_____ by _____ .

(% participation)   (date)

Method: I will accomplish increased participation of my staff in our shared governance council by:

_____

_____

_____

Accountability: I will measure my unit's shared governance participation by:

_____

_____

_____

HOLDING PEERS ACCOUNTABLE

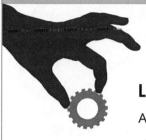

Learning Objectives

After reading this chapter, the participant will be able to:

✓ Examine how to promote accountability among peers

✓ Discuss conversation techniques for holding peers accountable

Accountability Conversations with Peers

The nature of an accountability culture and the dynamics of an effective accountability conversation are clearest when peers are involved. Here there is no clear line of authority to provide you with context. It's you trying to get another person to help you when the person doesn't have to. It's the other person trying to get your support when you do not have to be involved.

The fact that all parties are equal puts the focus on the nature of the relationship you are creating. Most accountability conversations are about building relationships. Trust has to be built and communication has to be effective. Accountability is relationship-driven; it's about relationships without fear of blame or punishment.

Who are your peers?

Think about who your peers are. If you are a staff nurse, your peers are fellow staff nurses and anyone with whom you may be working side by side. They are the pharmacists and lab technicians you often interact with. If you are a nurse manager, your peers are the other nurse managers or managers of other departments. If you are a director or vice president, they are the other directors and vice presidents.

Peers are the people who are at your level within the organization. You find yourself interacting with them, often on matters that affect your performance or your unit's performance. Imagine situations where you needed to have a peer do something beyond his or her day-to-day duties in order for you to succeed. Consider these examples:

- As a nurse manager, you need another nurse manager to assist you by floating staff members to your unit

- As a nurse on the floor, you need to reorganize the work flow with the other nurses to ensure that everyone on the shift gets an appropriate meal break

- As a vice president or director, you need the information systems and HR departments to join you in a new change initiative that will require them to perform in a different way

Having the conversation

You need to make sure the environment you create is free of punishment and blame and allows people to take risks. You need to make requests and offers. You need to ask your peers to make commitments and find out what it may take for them to keep their commitments.

Remember, commitments need to be defined, measurable, and time-limited. When you are dealing with other people—in this situation, a peer—you need to make sure you understand what the expectations are, the person you are working with understands what the expectations are, and you do your part to create an environment that supports and demands accountability.

There are two types of peer accountability conversations. One is where the peer can say "yes" because it's already part of his or her work or ability. Here the attention is on clear communication. You can generally expect a "yes."

Here are some examples:

- As a new nurse, you need to ask your preceptor to show you a procedure that you have never done before

- As a nurse manager, you ask the HR manager to assist you with a disciplinary action conversation with a member of your staff

The other type of peer accountability conversation is where the request you make may seem to be disruptive to the peer's work and schedule. Here you need to enroll the person in your initiative. Think of the conversation as having three stages: creating readiness, crafting the commitment, and acknowledging delivery of the commitment.

Stage 1: Creating readiness

Before you make the request, you want the person to be ready to hear it in a positive mindset. You may have to build up readiness by having a series of conversations.

Conversation for relatedness:	Show how together you have a common mission
Conversation for possibility:	Surface a future state that excites your peer
Conversation for opportunity:	Show how the current situation can benefit from a joint effort and that both parties can make it work
Conversation for commitment:	Make the request and offer

Creating readiness is creating a relationship with the other person. You are seeking a partnership. You are asking yourself: What does it take to get a commitment from this person? It comes down to how you need to "be." How do you need to "be" in the moment to attract the other person? Here are some examples of creating readiness.

☑ ACCOUNTABILITY SPOTLIGHT

Staff nurse

As a staff nurse, you frequently find that the medication cart is messy and not stocked (people use things in the cart and do not replace them). You would like to organize the cart so that things are easier to find, and create a process that nurses restock their carts at the end of their shifts. You know that the condition of the medication cart bothers another nurse on your unit. This nurse works a schedule similar to yours. You would like this nurse to assist you in this project.

You engage this nurse in a conversation about your frustration with the medication cart. This nurse agrees with you (common mission). You explain that you think there is a way to reorganize the cart and then have each nurse restock the cart at the end of his or her shift. You show her a diagram you made of the cart, reorganized to make it easier to find things. You ask her for her input (possibility and opportunity). You ask her whether she would be willing to try it with you (make the request).

Manager

As a manager, you know your unit stocks only 1000ml bottles of normal saline and sterile water. You notice that nurses discard bottles that are more than half full because they have not been used within 24 hours. You contact the manager of materials management and highlight this situation. You inquire about the availability and cost of 500ml bottles. The smaller bottles could be less expensive and easier to store, which are two issues you know your materials management peer is addressing throughout the hospital (common mission and joint benefit). The materials management manager lets you know that 500ml bottles are available and would cost less. The storage shelf on your unit will need to be slightly reorganized to fit the necessary number of smaller bottles. You ask the manager to make the change to the 500ml bottles (make the request).

Stage 2: Crafting commitment

When you reach the point of making commitments you need to do the following:

- Make requests and offers

- Actively listen

- Ask the partners what it would take for them to meet their commitments

- Use DNA to capture the interest already there:

  - Define what you want

  - Notice it when you get it

  - Acknowledge/celebrate it

- Capture the commitment in writing with all the critical elements

For example, when you and the other staff nurse have successfully reorganized the medication cart and tested the new process by having three nurses, one on each shift, restock the cart at the end of their shift, you put up a sign in the staff lounge announcing the project and acknowledging those who have been part of the work. You invite other nurses to try the process. For those who do not embrace the new process, you publicly ask them why not as well as what it would take for them to try the new process. You listen for them to make an offer of participation. You have to be willing to listen to and hear a suggestion of how to make the process better for others.

For the materials management manager who helped you stock the 500ml bottles of normal saline and sterile water on your unit, you look for a way to publicly thank this manager and celebrate your joint success. Perhaps it is at your hospital's next managers' meeting. You announce the project that you worked on and acknowledge the success, which was made possible by the materials management manager who was willing to work with you.

Stage 3: Acknowledging delivery of commitments

A commitment always has a delivery date. It's always clear that the commitment is either delivered or not delivered. Interestingly, both situations are positive and call for celebration. With delivery, the celebration is about results. Without delivery, the celebration is about learning and renewed commitment.

We have all been in that difficult circumstance where someone doesn't keep to a commitment, or doesn't do what he or she committed to doing.

This can mean that one of the following three situations occurred:

1. The person did not really commit upfront. We did not listen carefully.

2. The person did commit, and then forgot about it. The person did not act.

3. The person did commit. The person tried. What he or she tried did not work out.

In an accountability culture, it is always appropriate to discuss which of the three is driving the current situation.

Situation #1 opens up the accountability conversation again. Go through the readiness and crafting steps. This time, listen better for the "yes/no." For example, when working with the other nurse to reorganize the medication cart, you have come up with a new way to organize the drawers and she tells you she will keep the drawers organized like this "when she can." After two weeks, you notice that her cart is not kept in the way you had agreed. You did not hear the "when she can," which was her lack of commitment.

For the materials management manager, you reviewed how your storage area would be reorganized to accommodate the smaller bottles of normal saline and sterile water. The manager tells you the shelves will be reorganized "as soon as we can." Three weeks later, the shelves have still not been reorganized. You did not hear the "as soon as we can," which was the lack of commitment. You could have avoided both situations with one question: "Will you commit to try to keep the medication drawers organized in this way for three weeks?" or "By what date will the storage shelves be reorganized?"

Situation #2 requires that the person clean up the mess. Acknowledge the shortfall in performance and recommit to action. This is a teaching moment about trust and partnership.

For example, when the staff nurse does not restock the cart at the end of her shift, you approach her about the commitment she made and ask her what challenges she encountered in keeping the commitment. She acknowledges that she got busy and forgot to do it at the end of two shifts this week. You listen for a "request" to revise her commitment and you ask for a new commitment, which will include a measurable result by a specified time.

When you notice that your shelves have not been stocked with the 500ml sterile water and normal saline, you contact the materials management manager who tells you that he delegated the task to someone else and forgot to follow up to see that it was done as agreed. He apologizes and promises that it will be completed by Friday.

Situation #3 is a success in that something was intentionally tried and learning has occurred. Now you can build the next commitments on that learning.

For example, the staff nurse tells you that on shifts when she has had two or more admissions, it is impossible for her to restock the medication cart before she leaves. The two of you review the process and agree to try another way to keep the commitment: You will try asking the nurse coming on duty to stock the cart before she starts her rounds with patients. You agree to track this and expect that it will occur only when a nurse has had two or more admissions on a shift.

When the materials management manager tells you that he can get 500ml bottles of normal saline, but he cannot get sterile water for about two months, you agree to make the change to the 500ml bottles of normal saline and wait for the 500ml bottles of sterile water to be available in two months. In two months, you check back with the manager.

We are always producing results and getting smarter. It's not about blame; it's not about punishment. It's about finding out what it would take for people to keep their commitments.

The Power of Public Accountability

It is important to realize that most of your accountability conversations happen in public. They happen in meetings with a lot of other people. Although it is still important to have one-on-one conversations, most of your opportunities will be "in the moment" conversations as part of team or group meetings. Get used to it. Look for these opportunities to engage your peers in your objectives. All of this happens in public. That's why it is an accountability culture.

Another tool that is often effective when working with peers is a public declaration—getting someone to make a commitment publicly. There are amazing benefits to this. When conversations with peers result in a public commitment, a lot of positive things happen. It's sort of an amplification tool; it amplifies the commitment. For many people, it also helps them to understand that the commitment they made is a promise and something on which they need to follow through. A public declaration of commitment by a peer also allows you to enroll others more easily.

Let's look at an example of how you can be in an accountability conversation with peers to secure the commitments you need.

☑ ACCOUNTABILITY SPOTLIGHT

I was in a meeting recontly with nursing managers and HR managers. We were a team of about 15 people working on a new hiring system to solve a staff shortage problem. With the system, called *predictive hiring*, we anticipate turnover and recruit in advance to keep vacancies close to zero. In the meeting, we were mapping out the work to be done and seeking commitments from all parties about what they were going to do differently to deliver for this new process.

We knew that for us to get ahead of our vacancy issue, we needed to deal with two issues. One was to have a certain number of hires each month to account for turnover. The other was to institute an extraordinary hiring effort for several months to fill a number of vacancies that had accumulated over time. We had done our homework and we knew what those hires needed to be.

We asked our HR manager whether he could commit to making that number of hires each month. This would require the HR department to recruit and hire way beyond its natural monthly performance.

In response, the manager talked about the activity involved, but did not say "yes." He understood why we needed to fill those positions in that period of time, but he was cautious. He was hesitant to make the commitment.

In the conversation, one had to listen carefully to realize the response was a "yes, but." It was, in effect, "yes, we will do the best we can . . . yes, we agree it's important, but it's unlikely we can perform at that level." This is a very natural response. He was excited about the project. He wanted it to succeed. But all of a sudden he was being asked to commit to an effort that appeared to him to be well beyond his reach. We all are trained to respond to a request like this with a "no" and do it in a nice way. That nice, polite way often makes it hard to hear the "no."

It is important to hear this natural response as a "no" and, in doing so, to avoid any negative judgment about the person. (There is no blame in an accountability culture.) All that has happened is that I have made a request and he has not said "yes" yet.

We continued the conversation. We asked him what it would take for him to make that commitment. What were his concerns? He told us he was afraid that if he made the commitment and didn't deliver on it, he would let everyone down. He was afraid he would be setting himself up for punishment or blame.

As a team, we had to have a conversation about the nature of the commitment being requested. The request was beyond the reach of his current practice. It was also clear that by turning to the team for help, we all could put in place activities that would create the desired results. We were a team. We needed him to make a commitment to the bold goal and we also needed to create a supportive environment where he could ask for the help he needed. He could say to us, "To make this many hires in a month, I'm going to need help to do these things."

By having the goal, he can now come to us and make requests and offers. We need him to stand for that recruiting goal for the team. We need to work with him to achieve the team's goals.

☑ **ACCOUNTABILITY SPOTLIGHT**

In another example, I am talking with a peer about a challenge they are facing. They tell me about how they need help from nursing to resolve a problem.

I was trying to get him to make a request of me, something that we could work on together to help with this problem. It was obviously of great concern to him. One of the questions that I asked him was, "What worries you most about this problem and working with nursing to address?" He told me what his worry was and then I turned that around and said, "I will make a commitment to you. I hear your concern.*

Now, can we identify something else that nursing can do to help you with this problem?"

*You need nurses on the units to do _____. I will work with the nurse managers to have the nurses do _____. I will monitor that the nurses do what we said.

My commitment to him made it safe for him to make additional requests of me. He knew that he could count on me to deliver what I told him I would deliver.

Holding your peers accountable can be hard. You work together, you like each other, and you don't want to jeopardize relationships. These are the exact reasons why you NEED to hold your peers accountable. You would want them to do the same for you. Not holding them accountable hurts you as much as it does them. This is not about blame, punishment, or bad stories. Healthcare is hard work. We need each other to be successful.

Holding each other accountable is just how we need to be. I have given you the techniques and tools . . . give them a try.

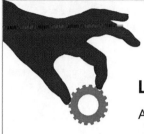

CHAPTER 6

SEEKING ACCOUNTABILITY FROM YOUR MANAGER

Learning Objectives

After reading this chapter, the participant will be able to:

✓ Assess the level of accountability of your manager or supervisor

✓ Determine methods to promote accountability from your manager or supervisor

Managing Up

We have talked about the tools for accountability and how they relate to personal accountability, and then we talked about how to hold your peers accountable.

What about managing up? How do you hold your manager or supervisor accountable? Remember, accountability is about commitments. It's doing what you say you are going to do. To get your manager or supervisor to be accountable, you use the same accountability tools you used in the other situations: your personal accountability and holding your staff and peers accountable.

Start with language

It starts with the language you use. Remember, it's the "yes" or "no." Ask for a commitment and hear the "no," which may be phrased as a "yes, but."

In previous chapters, we talked about requests, offers, declarations, and assertions. This is the language you use. Ask (request) for the commitment you want. If you don't hear the commitment you want, offer to help achieve the commitment. You can use the same skills even if the person with whom you are communicating is your manager or supervisor.

☑ ACCOUNTABILITY SPOTLIGHT

Let's look at an example of how this might work. Let's say you are a nurse having problems on your unit with people being on time to start their shift. The staff members who come on duty to relieve you are frequently a few minutes late, which delays you in giving report and finishing your shift. You think your manager should hold staff members accountable.

You have a conversation with your manager and share your concerns. The manager agrees with you, noting that recently this seems to be an increasing problem. She tells you she intends to address it at next week's staff meeting. You are concerned that this will not be enough to change the problem. You can ask (make a request) your manager how she will measure the improvement in the behavior. If she does not suggest (offer) anything to be measured, you can suggest (make an offer) that she monitor staff members reporting to work on time for four weeks. If there is no improvement, you can suggest (make a request) that something else be done. If your manager says "no" to any of your requests, modify them so that she can say "yes."

How do you get people to make commitments, and in particular, how do you get them to keep those commitments? Sometimes what sounds like a lack of commitment just needs to be restated in such a way that the commitment can be met.

The other tool we talked about using is stopping and resetting. When you are in an encounter with your manager and supervisor and you are not hearing accountability, you can always stop the conversation and reset its context. It's important that your conversations remain effective. Remember, we talked about effective listening: Listen to understand. It may mean stopping a negative conversation and resetting the conversation so that a commitment can be made. Accountability language does work!

* Definition of bad story: a technique used by many, often unconsciously, to defend against change. Bad stories are usually based on someone's perception of past performance and may have limited basis in fact. Sometimes they are just a way to "vent," which can be okay. In an accountability culture, bad stories need to be called for what they are and should not be allowed to prevent accountability from occurring.

Reset the conversation

When trying to reset a conversation, effective questions are helpful. One effective question is "What worries you?" Asking your supervisor what is preventing him or her from making a commitment, and most especially, from keeping that commitment, is critical.

It also may mean some difficult conversations. It means not being afraid to ask questions. You need to be cautious when you hear negativity, or when you're making a negative judgment about someone not making a commitment. It requires you to understand why the person can't make the commitment and how the commitment could be restated or revised.

For example, as a nurse manager, you have an idea for a new staffing model for your unit. You discuss the model with your director. The director's response to your idea is lukewarm. You hear "yes, but . . ." or maybe even a "no."

You know you need a commitment of support, so you respond, "I sense hesitation. What worries you about my plan?"

The director explains his concern about your ability to meet productivity expectations with your model.

You respond, "I understand that you are not sure my model will allow me to meet productivity expectations. I have tested the model. Can I show you how the model will work so that I can meet productivity expectations? I am committed to meeting the productivity expectations. Can I try my model for one schedule so that I can demonstrate this?"

When you request a commitment, what response is this person making? When you hear "yes, but . . ." that's really a "no" for the commitment. You can turn that "yes, but . . ." into a true "yes" by hearing it as a request for help and being able to respond to that request with an offer.

Set the scene

When you deal with a manager or a supervisor, you should also be thinking about another tool. We talked about it earlier when we discussed flipping the work or flipping the energy. Supervisors or managers have two ways of thinking. One is administrative mode—getting the work done, paying attention to details, and zooming in. Some may even call it micromanaging.

The other is leadership mode: being able to make goals, to think about something that is larger than the situation at hand.

Often, we find that a manager or supervisor is spending his or her time in administrative mode wanting to make sure we pay attention to details and that we get our job done. He or she seems to discourage risks or discourages people from thinking bigger. When you think about that manager or supervisor who is not accountable, how are you hearing that person talking to you? What work is he or she talking about doing?

For example, you would like to create an initiative to improve a process in your hospital. You know it will have to be an interdisciplinary group. You are not really sure of the solution, but you believe that if you get the right people together, the process can be measurably improved. You discuss your idea with your manager. Immediately, your manager starts telling you how to fix the problem, even though he is not involved in the actual process. Rather than hearing this as a "no," you can flip it to an offer: "I'm glad you agree that this process is a problem. Thank you for your offer to help us improve it. Can I include you in the team I will assemble to fix the process?"

Your manager responds, "I don't think I need to be on your team. Just make sure you look at the things I mentioned."

End result: You have support to create your team and some process improvement suggestions to include.

When I walk into a management meeting, a senior management meeting for that matter, I have to listen for what's happening in the meeting and think about how I am going to "be" in that meeting. I do this before every meeting I attend. What is the "work" of the meeting? Is it administrative or leadership in nature?

Whether it's a large group or a one-on-one meeting, I need to understand why I'm in the meeting and what is being expected of me. What kind of work is being done?

I may be asked to attend a meeting where a problem needs to be solved. This will require me to understand details and participate in the performance improvement. This is administrative or supervisory work. If I were to come into that meeting with ideas about how the organization should look forward and think about things that are larger than this particular problem, people in the meeting (perhaps even my manager or supervisor) may wonder what I'm trying to do or what the conversation is about. The work at hand is administrative. It's getting this problem fixed.

From a leadership role, if I'm being brought into a conversation with my manager or supervisor or if I'm in a meeting with some senior executives and we are trying to chart a course for the organization or trying to be strategic, that's leadership work. If I came into that meeting and got caught in the details of every suggestion that was made, I would be trying to administrate that issue and would not be a leader in that role. I would create negative energy in the room and interrupt the work at hand.

It is important that when you hear a manager or a supervisor not being accountable, you think about how he or she is looking at the work. Is it administrative or leadership work? How can you get your manager/supervisor to be in the role you need him or her to be in?

Once you understand the work at hand and how your manager/supervisor is viewing the work, you can use some of the tools we have discussed to get him or her to "be" in the right kind of work.

- Make requests and offers

- Ask effective questions

- Stop, reset

Flip negative energy

Negative energy can also show up in other ways. We have all been in the situation where we are talking with a manager or supervisor about something and what we hear are all the reasons our idea won't work.

We may hear:

"Oh, we tried that here a couple of years ago and that's just not going to happen here"

or

"Oh, yes, I think that's a great idea but that's just not going to work here"

or

"Do you remember so-and-so? He tried that here and he doesn't work here anymore"

When we walk away from that conversation we feel defeated. We feel shot down. We need to think about how we can respond to the negative energy.

How do you flip negative energy to positive energy? In that conversation, when your manager or supervisor is telling you why something won't work it's important to ask questions.

- Find out

- Listen to understand

- What are your manager or supervisor's concerns?

Your response could be:

> *"I didn't know we had tried this here before. Can you tell me more about how it was done and, in your opinion, why it didn't work?"*

As you listen to understand, you can make a request or you can make an offer:

> *"I hear you say that when this was tried before it didn't work for these reasons. Well, I'd like to make an offer. I would like to try it this way. Here is how I think my suggestion will be different from the first attempt . . ."*

You are making an offer to elicit a commitment, to elicit accountability. Fashion the offer so that your manager/supervisor *can* make a commitment.

Pacing event

Another tool you can use to hold your manager or supervisor accountable is a pacing event. A pacing event is a forum for public displays of accountability and public commitments. It's much easier to have people keep to a commitment when they have publicly declared it. Sometimes a pacing event can be an effective tool to use with a manager or supervisor when you aren't sure that you really have a commitment.

It means talking with your manager or supervisor about an idea, something you would like to do, and for which you want his or her commitment or support. Your manager or supervisor tells you "yes" and you hear, "yes, but . . ." So, you make an offer and now that "yes, but . . ." sounds more like a "yes."

You can introduce the idea of a pacing event. It means saying to your manager or supervisor, "I'm really excited about what we are talking about doing here. I would like to bring it up in our next staff meeting so that we can announce to everyone else in the department what we are doing about this. I think we can get some great energy around it and I think we can get some people engaged." That's a pacing event—when you make that public declaration, that public display of accountability and commitment.

Dealing with Different Types of Managers

Now that we have talked a little bit about the tools you can use with your manager or supervisor to get some accountability, let's think a bit more about different types of managers or supervisors you might encounter.

Don't-make-waves manager

Some managers or supervisors have the motto "Keep your head down. Do your work and don't make any waves." I once had a job where the manager's motto was "Keep our name out of the newspaper." The manager avoided commitments, especially anything beyond direct responsibility.

Remember we talked about the differences between responsibility and accountability: Responsibility means getting things to respond to you, and accountability means taking account for actions.

When managers or supervisors say:

> *"Keep your head down, do your work, don't make any waves, don't take any risks, don't go out there on that limb,"*

it's important to *listen to understand*. What are they afraid of? What's preventing them from being able to make a commitment? How do you turn that *"yes, but . . ."* or what might really be a *"no"* into a commitment? What would it take for them to be able to make that commitment? I often use the expression, *"What's it going to take for your manager or supervisor to make a commitment today?"*

You may work through your requests and offers to come up with a commitment that can be made. Remember, it may not be the commitment you were looking for; it may be something less, but a commitment is still a commitment. It's a step in the right direction. For people who aren't accepting accountability, a commitment that is made, that they can keep, and that they can follow through on is a move in the right direction to getting them accountable.

Promises-the-world manager

Let's talk about another kind of manager or supervisor you might encounter: the one who promises the world but then doesn't deliver. You hear great ideas and commitments, but then you don't see any action. You feel like you are accountable but your manager is not. So, what do you do in that situation?

When you hear someone making commitments and you know his or her behavior is to not follow through on those commitments, use the accountability tools we discussed. Remember, when you are talking in accountability terms, you need to be specific. You need to define what you want. You need to be realistic. The commitment needs to be measurable and time-limited. When someone is making big promises you know he or she won't or can't keep, it's important for you to listen and to ask questions. Ensure that the commitment is defined, measurable, and time-limited. You will need to make requests and offers.

For example, when you hear someone making promises you know will not be delivered, ask very specific questions about the commitment. What exactly will that person deliver? If you don't feel it's realistic, what request can you make to make it more realistic? Is it measurable? How will you know when the commitment happens or, more importantly, doesn't happen? As a time limit, do you know when you can expect the commitment to be achieved? In this situation, it's important to follow up, whether through e-mail or via a conversation, to confirm the commitment you heard. It is very important to ensure that you follow up if the person has not met the commitment by the time limit.

It's like being in a meeting or on a committee where everyone sits down to tackle a problem and lots of people are nodding their heads, indicating that they agree this is the right approach. You leave the meeting feeling good that you have a plan that's going to work. Six months later you're back in that same meeting, wondering why you're trying to solve the same problem again. Those situations occur because no one defined the commitment. Define what you want. Make sure it's realistic. Make sure it's measurable and time-limited. Provide follow-up to ensure that the commitment was met. If the commitment was not met, the person is not "off the hook." You need to revise the commitment in defined, measurable, time-limited terms. Throw in a little "public declaration" so that others join you in holding the person accountable!

Remember, the other effective tool to use for managers who aren't accountable is DNA:

- Define what you want

- Notice it when you get it

- Acknowledge it or celebrate it

So, whether it's the manager who tells you to keep your head down and just do your work without making any waves and without accepting accountability, or the manager who promises the world and doesn't deliver, use DNA. Define what you want, notice it when you get it, acknowledge it, and celebrate it because you are trying to reinforce that behavior.

How It Feels to Be Held Accountable

Here are a few more examples of situations I've been in where either I as the manager or supervisor have been held accountable by the folks I work with, or I have used accountability as an effective tool with my manager or supervisor.

☑ ACCOUNTABILITY SPOTLIGHT

At our hospital, one of our nurse managers was engaging in a project that would affect departments across the hospital. She had engaged people to work with her on this project. They had all made commitments and were accepting accountability for things that were beyond their direct responsibility. She wanted my help to make sure people across the organization could understand the project. By lending my name and support to the project, she was hoping she would help to keep people on track and allow them to keep the commitments they had made. She asked me to make a commitment. She told me she needed me to take a specific event and a specific action at a certain time and location. She then asked me whether I could commit to do it. I told her I could; the day before I was to do what she had asked me to commit to, she sent me a reminder e-mail stating, "Remember that tomorrow is the day and here is what I need you to do." It was defined, realistic, measurable, and time-limited. Again, at the end of her e-mail she asked me whether I could keep the commitment. That's how she was holding me accountable.

Another time I was working with our chief operating officer (COO). We were working on a project that was going across the organization. I knew I would have to have senior leadership approval and support, so I went to my immediate supervisor who suggested that I go to the COO.

I went to the COO, explained the project, and asked whether he could commit to and support what we were doing. I had to explain what was being done that was different. I had to let him know what the measurable outcomes were going to be. I explained how I thought the individual departments would be affected. I asked whether he could make a commitment. His response was "yes, but . . ." I restated what I thought was his concern because I thought. I heard him say, "Yes, I am committed to the project, but I have a concern." So, I asked him what worried him about the project. He told me his concerns, and I restated them so that he could affirm that I heard correctly. Then I made a commitment that those problems would not occur, that I would accept the accountability for his concern not becoming a reality. He then was able to make the commitment. He was able to say "yes" and was able to help me communicate about the project.

I have given you a couple of examples of the kinds of managers or supervisors you may encounter who don't appear to be accountable, and how you can help them become accountable. I have also given you some examples that I have encountered as a manager or supervisor. Now it's time to talk about how to make physicians accountable, something we'll tackle in the next chapter.

PHYSICIANS AND ACCOUNTABILITY

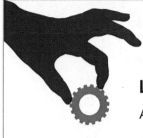

Learning Objectives

After reading this chapter, the participant will be able to:

✓ Examine accountability challenges nurses face with physicians

✓ Determine how to define expectations

✓ Explain how to set commitments

✓ List words to use when interacting with physicians

Language Tools

In previous chapters, we talked about how to achieve accountability—in ourselves, our peers, and our managers and supervisors. Now, let's talk about physicians.

We have many opportunities to work with physicians. It may be in caring for a specific patient or group of patients, or we may work with them on a project or team. Working with physicians to achieve accountability is no different from working with anyone else. We want to get physicians to do what they say they are going to do. We want them to make commitments and keep their commitments.

We will use the same tools we used earlier. We'll start with the language we use. We want to use the six language tools we discussed in Chapter 2. The format is the same as covered in Chapter 2, but with physician specifics:

1. **Framing:** Turn on the listening you need

2. **Effective questions:** Turn on the physician's creative power

3. **Active listening:** Make sure the physician is being heard and understood

4. **Requests and offers:** Generate commitments

5. **Hear yes/no:** Verify accountability

6. **Acknowledgment:** Celebrate behavior that works

1. Framing

Framing an accountability conversation is how you "set the stage" for what is expected. Often, you don't achieve the results you desire because the expectations were not clear or each party had different expectations. Framing allows you to define what you expect.

Framing is when you ask the physician to listen and process in a positive way. It creates the listening opportunity for you to speak. It creates one common mindset in the conversation and enables participants to do the correct work.

You can easily fix the mindset in a conversation or meeting by asking people to be a certain way, to do a specific kind of work, and to be open to the possibility of accountability.

In a group conversation involving physicians, framing sounds like this:

- I'm asking everyone to be in a leadership role for this session

- I ask us to focus on our vision of improving our patient satisfaction scores by five percentage points in six months

- I ask us to listen to the presentation for opportunities we can pursue to make progress on our goal

- Please be prepared to make commitments at the end, thank you

You can do the same thing in a one-on-one conversation with a physician. For example, let's say you are caring for a patient in pain. You contact the physician and use the SBAR technique (situation background assessment recommendation) to communicate the patient's condition. You confer with the physician about how reasonable pain control can be achieved, and the physician gives you an order for pain medicine. You commit to the physician that you will give the medication as ordered and you will call the physician in three hours if the patient's pain has not improved (pain level < 5) for further orders. The physician agrees with the plan.

Everyone wants to do the right work and to contribute. All we have to do is ask!

2. Effective questions

Effective questions can be very helpful in achieving accountability. These questions focus on what is working and how effective activities and outcomes can be replicated. They generate positive energy and possibilities. They require that you understand another person's position.

Effective questions are a valuable tool to use in a group setting, such as a meeting. In a meeting, you want participants to process information in a useful way that adds value. However, all of the people in the room are asking themselves questions and continually answering them. By setting the questions for them, you can make the meeting much more productive.

Here's how it works. You are describing a proposed plan to improve operating room turnover times. As you are speaking, the three questions in people's minds are:

1. What is wrong with this proposal?

2. Why won't this work?

3. Should I support this?

These questions will likely produce negative, highly critical responses. They take the energy out of the room. The response back could be defensive.

To create a more productive response, before you speak give the audience the effective questions you want them to address (framing) as they listen to the proposal to improve turnover times in the operating room.

For example:

- What works?

- What do you find exciting?

- How does this contribute to our goals?

- What would you add to make it better?

These are "effective questions" in that they generate positive insights and additions. They are generative; they can't be answered with a yes or no.

3. Active listening

Listening can be a passive activity. As you are listening, you can be distracted, superimposing your own thoughts, drifting.

Listening is work. In active listening, the listener restates in is or her own language what he or she heard the speaker say and his or her impression of what the speaker said. The speaker can then confirm that what was heard was what he or she intended. If it wasn't, the speaker can restate what he or she said. This can continue until the speaker confirms that he or she has been "heard."

Active listening is hard. You have to really listen to what is being said and confirm what you intend people to hear. Active listening gives proof that the listener has understood the speaker. Another advantage of active listening is that it keeps responsibility for solving problems with the speaker. If you do not understand what the speaker is intending, it is the speaker's responsibility to explain.

Accountability means doing what you say you are going to do. Often, a lack of accountability is due to miscommunication and unmet expectations. If we are going to hold people accountable, we need to ensure that they have heard the expectation and we have heard the commitment to meet the expectation.

In your conversations and meetings, frequently ask participants, "What is being said? What are you hearing?"

4. Requests and offers

How many times have you talked about what you needed but not received a response from the person you were talking to or meeting with? We are good at describing and explaining. We are not good at asking.

Requests and offers are one of the most powerful speech acts available to us. This is how you generate commitments. You make requests, you make offers. Most meetings do not end with people leaving in action, because no one made a request and offer. It was assumed that everyone knew what to do.

At some point in the meeting, stop to make requests and offers. You can give each person an opportunity to speak. When responding to a request or offer, you have two choices: You can say "yes" or you can say "no." If you say "no," it helps to make a counteroffer. A "no" is often the beginning of a longer conversation.

When you hear a "no," you may need to make a request or an offer. Your request will sound like, "What would it take for you to say yes?" This reminds me of the last time I bought a car and the dealer asked me, "What would it take for you to buy this car today?" He was asking me to make a commitment.

5. Yes/no

When you are talking to someone about accountability, you are often asking a simple question: "Are you accountable?" You want to know whether this person is committed to achieving the result under discussion. Too often we hear what we want to rather than what was said.

Yes/no is about listening for the "yes" or "no." People rarely answer accountability questions with a "yes" or "no." They talk. We mistake talking for a commitment. We mistake nodding of heads to be a commitment. We mistake "yes, but . . ." for a "yes."

You have to develop an ear for the response. Active listening helps here. "I am hearing you say that you cannot accept accountability right now because . . . Is that correct?"

6. Acknowledgment

We have walked through steps that can surface commitments and the content and energy that lead to commitments. To get more accountability you have to acknowledge it when it happens.

Too often we see accountability and almost dismiss it as "someone just doing his or her job." If you are successful in getting someone to make a commitment and most importantly to keep that commitment, you need to acknowledge and celebrate it.

In his book *Enlightened Leadership*, Doug Krug talks about a version of this practice which he calls DNA. To get more of what you want, use DNA:

- Define what you want.

- Notice it when you get it.

- Acknowledge/celebrate it.

☑ **ACCOUNTABILITY SPOTLIGHT**

I had the opportunity to work with a new medical director in one of our procedural areas. He was very excited about making some changes in the department to improve patient outcomes. His first intention was to make the changes and send out a memo to his colleagues and the staff announcing the changes. We discussed potential barriers to this approach. He revised his approach and instead reviewed the changes with his colleagues and the staff for their input and feedback. After incorporating the input, he sent out the memo announcing that the changes would be effective in two weeks.

We celebrated the success of his approach at a division meeting.

In another situation, we were engaging a medical director in our negotiations with a vendor. This was a new approach for us. We educated the physician on our past negotiation practices as we had not included the physician in negotiations. We thought that we could improve our pricing if the physician participated in the negotiation process with us (defined what we wanted). He was very interested in working with us. The physician worked with us and we were able to save a significant amount of money. We celebrated this physician at an operations leadership and board-level meeting (noticed and celebrated).

In essence, you are rewarding/acknowledging the behavior you want to see and the individual is being positively reinforced.

You need to make sure that when you talk about commitments and ask physicians to make commitments, you ask a yes or no question. Are they able to make a commitment? What is the commitment they are making? You also need to be mindful of requests and offers. What requests can you make? What offers can you make to a physician in trying to help him or her achieve accountability? In addition, you may use declarations or assertions. Effective conversations are also key to helping physicians achieve accountability.

Furthermore, you need to use active listening and effective questions. What would it take for a physician to say yes to a commitment? What requests do you need to make to help a physician achieve accountability?

Listen to Understand

Now, we have talked about the language we can use and how we can be effective communicators. We also need to make sure we pay attention to active listening. We need to *listen to understand*.

An effective tool you can use in one-on-one conversations, and especially in groups, is to "stop and reset." I often think of it as a "timeout." In fact, when I'm in a group of people I know, I sometimes make a *T* with my hands and say, "Stop, timeout." I use the timeout as an opportunity to reset the energy in the room, essentially the tone of the conversation.

Another effective tool is to assess the energy in the room or in a conversation. You know what this feels like. Think about a meeting you have been in where there is energy and engagement—it feels like the land of possibility. Contrast that to the meeting you have been in where there is negative energy—all of the reasons why what you are discussing won't work. This can suck the life out of the room (and you!).

When you are in an accountability conversation, you need to assess the energy level. Positive energy is about what you can do. Negative energy is about what you cannot do. Net backward energy, according to Doug Krug, is where there are more negatives than positives; more about what you can't do than what you can do. Net forward energy, according to Krug, is about what can be done.

Rather than talking about what can't work or won't work, you need to talk about possibilities. You need to be able to focus on how you can flip negative energy. You also need to focus on the work at hand. Are you talking about administration of something or are you talking about leadership work? You need to make sure you are setting the right context for the work that needs to be done and that you are setting the right environment for achieving accountability, for making commitments, and most especially for keeping commitments.

One thing to note with physicians is communication style. Physicians are trained to be independent thinkers, to identify a problem and fix it. They often have a lesser level of comfort with "group thinking." Yet, in healthcare, we tend to use process improvement, performance improvement, and group thinking pretty often. We need to understand that we may be coming at a problem from different perspectives. We need to be willing to listen to understand when we are working with our physician partners.

One way to do that is to really understand the physicians' leadership story. What makes them tick? What is important to them? What do they value? Why do they do the job they are doing? It's important to take the time to understand that and to hear their leadership story.

Once you hear about someone's passion and what drives him or her, it makes it much easier for you to look for some common ground to establish a common place. You also need to listen effectively and actively. You need to listen to the voice you are speaking into. That really means to put yourself in the physician's shoes; to understand what's important from the physician's perspective.

Think about the language you use. You want to make sure you are pursuing and defining commitments. You want to define what you want. You want to make sure a commitment is definable, measurable, and time-limited.

Gaining physician accountability

Let's consider some of the situations you could encounter with physicians and how you can gain physician accountability.

For instance, say you are working with a physician on creating an order set or protocol. Often, physicians will leap to a solution. They know where they want to end up, so that is what they will push forward to achieve. They may not understand or acknowledge that the process involves others. In that situation, you need to understand where the physician is coming from, as well as the barriers he or she foresees. You need to work with the physician to define a process to see the possibilities and to ask what it would take for him or her to make a commitment to participate in developing the order set/protocol and then to follow the order set/protocol.

We worked closely with physicians in my organization regarding our compliance with verbal orders. We identified that our compliance—making sure verbal orders are signed, dated, and timed within a specified period—could be improved. We improved our compliance by defining physician and nurse accountability in the verbal order process. This understanding helped us to seek commitments.

First, we needed to define our verbal order process. We defined that a verbal order would be accepted only in an urgent situation and not for the sake of convenience. Then we needed the nurses to make that commitment. We made sure the nurses understood the regulations and requirements, and that they were accepting verbal orders only in urgent situations. We defined that as a nursing accountability; a commitment that nursing needed to make.

Next, we wanted to see what nursing could do to help physicians with their accountability. We worked with our health unit coordinators (HUCs) on the units to have them flag when a verbal order was written, to bring it to the physician's attention. We also talked about how the HUCs could identify verbal orders that were unsigned on a particular unit. Each HUC created a list on his or her unit that we put up in the physician's charting area; this list let the physicians know what charts on that unit had unsigned verbal orders.

We came up with several things nursing could do to bring verbal orders to the physicians' attention. As we went through the list, we also identified that nursing could do only so much, and that we needed to rely on physicians making the commitment to sign, date, and time their verbal orders within the specified period.

We created a monthly report of unsigned verbal orders by physician that we gave to the physician chiefs for follow-up.

We got to a place where we were able to differentiate between physician accountability and nurse accountability.

We drove the physician accountability by making sure the results we were expecting were definable, measurable, and time-limited. Then we used DNA for the physicians who improved their verbal order compliance. We defined what we wanted. We noticed it when we got it, and we acknowledged and celebrated it.

Sometimes, when working with a physician one on one, you may be trying to work through a problem to gain some accountability, while the physician is listing the reasons the plan you put in place won't work. Sometimes that one physician can be a little bit obstructive, particularly in a meeting where you are working through a process. As a result, the conversation is filled with a lot of negative energy.

That's where it's important that you call the "bad story,"* and then stop and reset the conversation. You must recognize that the physician isn't trying to cause trouble or obstruct your progress. The bad story may be the physician making a request for more information or a different approach. So, when you hear bad stories, you must not get caught up in the negative energy. You need to hear the concern being expressed and then make requests and offers to address that concern. You need to flip the negative energy, and ask effective questions so that you can come up with solutions that are part of the commitment that physicians can keep.

***Bad story:** A technique used by many, often unconsciously, to defend against change. Bad stories are usually based on someone's perception of past performance and may have limited basis in fact. Sometimes they are just a way to vent, which can be okay. In an accountability culture, they need to be called for what they are and should not be allowed to prevent accountability from occurring.*

I often encounter physicians with a concern. They tell me what the problem is, from their perspective. As a result, I may not get the whole story. It's important that in that situation I again use the tools of accountability. I effectively and actively listen to the concern the physician is bringing forward. I have to ask more effective questions of everyone involved to understand the true situation.

Once I have gathered the necessary information, I can seek commitments to improve the situation. I try to include all involved parties in my discussions. I validate what I learned and discuss solutions. As we work to implement solutions, I ask for commitments. I don't stop until I get those commitments—defined, measurable, and time-limited. I make requests, offers, declarations, and assertions. I also communicate how I will follow up to ensure that the commitments are kept.

When someone comes to me with a concern or an issue, I ask questions so that I can fully understand the situation. I may also ask the physician to make multiple smaller commitments before we get to the major commitment.

Recently I had a great physician accountability experience. We had been tackling Core Measures compliance, particularly with CHF – ACEI/ARB utilization documentation. We had implemented a process where nurses would identify a chart lacking ACEI/ARB documentation by flagging it for the physician. In addition, the nurse would call the physician to address the documentation. Each week, the nurse would report all documentation issues (opportunities for improvement) to our chiefs. We saw our compliance improve with this process.

However, I was getting concerned that we would need to continue this cumbersome process indefinitely. I was not sure we were affecting changes in behavior or holding individual physicians accountable.

Our hospitalists' medical director asked whether nursing could provide a spreadsheet, listing physicians with "opportunities for improvement" by week so that he could address individual physician performance. He asked nursing (made a request!) to help him hold physicians accountable for their Core Measures documentation!

When you think about how you hold physicians accountable, it's really no different from any other group we have talked about. It comes down to the language you use, the situation you create, and making sure the results you want are definable, measurable, and time-limited. It means you need to actively listen. It also means using the DNA tool: defining what you want, noticing it when you get it, and acknowledging and celebrating it when you see it.

I work with many excellent physicians. When don't hear them being accountable, I ask questions (make requests) so that I can understand what is preventing them from being accountable. I will ask them "what will it take for you to do ____?" I am often surprised that what they tell me IS something I can do and do for them.

Think about a physician you work with, maybe someone with whom you have a good relationship who could use some accountability help. Try using some of the approaches and tools I've discussed here. You will be surprised to see how easy it can be to improve their accountability. It is hard work, but stick with it and you will reap many dividends.

PROMOTING ACCOUNTABILITY WITH THE C-SUITE

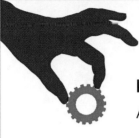

Learning Objectives

After reading this chapter, the participant will be able to:

✓ List effective words to use with C-suite members

✓ Describe how to establish common ground with C-suite members

✓ Discuss how your communication style enables C-suite accountability

Reaching Upward

We have talked about your personal accountability; we have talked about how to hold your peers accountable; we have talked about your manager and supervisor and how to get them to be accountable; and we have discussed how to achieve accountability with our physicians.

In this chapter, we will talk about the C-suite: the senior executives in our organization whose job title starts with the word *chief*. This includes titles such as chief executive officer, chief financial officer, chief information officer, chief medical officer, chief nursing officer, and chief nurse executive. To get them to be accountable, you can use the same tools we discussed for the other groups we talked about in the book. Once again, these are the tools outlined in Chapter 2, but with some C-suite specifics.

Language Tools

The first tools we'll use are the language tools you can use to speak in terms of accountability:

1. **Framing:** Turn on the listening you need

2. **Effective questions:** Turn on the senior executive's creative power

3. **Active listening:** Make sure the senior executive is being heard and understood

4. **Requests and offers:** Generate commitments

5. **Hear yes/no:** Verify accountability

6. **Acknowledgment:** Celebrate behavior that works

1. Framing

By framing an accountability conversation, you "set the stage" for what is expected. Often, you don't achieve the results you desire because the expectations weren't clear or each party had different expectations. Framing allows you to define what you expect.

Framing is when you ask your senior executive to listen and process in a positive way. It creates one common mindset in the conversation and enables participants to do the correct work.

You can easily fix the mindset in a conversation or meeting by asking people to be a certain way, to do a specific kind of work, and to be open to the possibility of accountability.

In a group, framing sounds like this:

- I would ask all of us to be in our leadership role for this session

- I ask us to be about our vision of improving our employee satisfaction in relation to visibility of senior executives by 10 percentage points over the next 12 months

- I ask us to listen to the presentation for opportunities we can pursue to make progress on our goal

- Please be prepared to make commitments at the end, thank you

You can do the same thing in a one-on-one conversation with a senior executive.

☑ ACCOUNTABILITY SPOTLIGHT

For example, I wanted to implement anticipatory hiring within nursing in our organization. Our nurse managers have a good understanding of their controllable and uncontrollable turnover. Often, they can predict vacancies four to six months in advance, and they can anticipate vacancies. Our time to fill a nursing vacancy can be up to four months, depending on the specialty area. Our practice was to post a vacancy when we had a resignation in hand. With our policy requiring two weeks' notice, this left a unit with an actual vacancy for up to four months. The burden of this vacancy on the unit was tremendous. I wanted nurse managers to be able to post positions "in anticipation" of a vacancy, based on their unit's turnover, current vacancies, and so forth.

I had to present my proposal to our chief operating officer. I framed the meeting by telling him I had a presentation on how to address our vacancy rate. I told him I needed him to hear a new approach to posting vacant positions to address our vacancy rate and nurse turnover. I asked him to listen for the possibilities. I told him I was going to be asking him to make a commitment.

He asked questions to understand what I was saying throughout my presentation. At the end, he was hesitant about making a commitment. I asked him, "What worries you about my proposal?" After some thought, he said, "I am concerned that if this is successful, you could end up hiring beyond our actual need and have a negative vacancy rate." After laughing together for a minute, I told him, "Let me live for just a short time with a negative vacancy rate!"

I told him, "I am committed to keeping nursing at 100% productivity. I will work with our HR and position control systems to ensure that this does not occur." He approved my proposal with the expectation that I would update him in six months on the progress we had made— essentially prove the effectiveness of anticipative hiring. He was holding me accountable to deliver on my commitments.

I got the commitment I needed, with clear, defined, measurable, and time-limited expectations. Everyone wants to do the right work and to contribute. All we have to do is ask!

2. Effective questions

Effective questions can be very helpful in achieving accountability. Effective questions focus on what is working and how effective activities and outcomes can be replicated. These questions generate positive energy and possibilities. They require one to understand another's position.

Effective questions are a valuable tool to use in a group setting, such as a meeting. In a meeting, you want participants to process information in a useful way that adds value. However, all of the people in the room are asking themselves a question and continually answering it. By setting that question for them, you can make the meeting much more productive.

Here's how it works. You are describing a proposed plan for senior executives rounding in the hospital. As you are speaking, the three questions in people's mind are:

- What is wrong with this proposal?

- Why won't this work?

- Should I support this?

These questions will likely produce negative, highly critical responses. They take the energy out of the room. The response back could be defensive.

To create a more productive response, before you speak give the audience the effective questions you want them to address (framing) as they listen to the proposal for senior executive rounding in the hospital.

For example:

- What works?

- What do you find exciting?

- What ways would this contribute to our goals?

- What would you add to make it better?

These are effective questions in that they generate positive insights and additions. They are generative; they can't be answered with a "yes" or "no."

3. Active listening

Listening can be a passive activity. As you are listening, you can be distracted, superimposing your own thoughts, drifting.

Listening is work. In active listening, the listener restates in his or her own language what he or she heard the speaker say and his or her impression of what the speaker said. The speaker can then confirm that what was heard was what he or she intended. If it wasn't, the speaker can restate what he or she said. This can continue until the speaker confirms that he or she has been "heard."

Recently, in one of our executive leadership meetings, our chief executive officer (CEO) expressed concern about our compliance performance with medication reconciliation. He talked about our performance and his expectations. He asked difficult questions of the executive team.

One of our leaders restated what the CEO had said, and added, "I hear you saying . . . You don't know who is accountable for this performance. Who is the senior leader accountable for our medication reconciliation process? Who is going to ensure that this performance improves?"

The CEO affirmed what was heard. The senior executive team then identified the one senior executive who was accountable for this performance. That senior executive committed to improve our performance.

Active listening is hard. You have to really listen to what is being said and confirm what you intend people to hear. Active listening gives proof that the listener has understood the speaker. Another advantage of active listening is that it keeps responsibility for solving problems with the speaker. If you do not understand what the speaker is intending, it is the speaker's responsibility to explain.

Accountability means doing what you say you are going to do. Often, a lack of accountability is due to miscommunication and unmet expectations. If you are going to hold someone accountable, you need to ensure that he or she has heard the expectation and you have heard the commitment to meet the expectation.

In your conversations and meetings, frequently ask participants, "What is being said? What are you hearing?"

4. Requests and offers

How many times have you talked about what you needed but not received a response from the person you were talking to or meeting with? We are good at describing and explaining. We are not good at asking.

Requests and offers are one of the most powerful speech acts available to us. This is how you generate commitments. You make requests, you make offers. Most meetings do not end with people leaving in action, because no one made a request and offer. It was assumed that everyone knew what to do.

At some point in the meeting, stop to make requests and offers. You can give each person an opportunity to speak. When responding to a request or an offer, you have two choices: You can say "yes" or you can say "no." If you say "no," it helps to make a counteroffer. A "no" is often the beginning of a longer conversation.

When you hear a "no," you may need to make a request or an offer. Your request will sound like, "What would it take for you to say yes?"

5. Yes/no

When you are talking to someone about accountability, you are often asking a simple question: "Are you accountable?" You want to know whether this person is committed to achieve the result under discussion. Too often we hear what we want to rather than what was said.

Yes/no is about listening for the "yes" or "no." People rarely answer accountability questions with a "yes" or "no." They talk. We mistake talking for a commitment. We mistake nodding of heads to be a commitment. We mistake hearing "yes, but . . ." for a "yes."

You have to develop an ear for the response. Active listening helps here. *"I am hearing you say that you cannot accept accountability right now because . . . Is that correct?"*

6. Acknowledgment

To get more accountability, you have to acknowledge it when it happens. Too often, we see accountability and almost dismiss it as "someone just doing his or her job." If you are successful in getting someone to make a commitment and, most importantly, keep that commitment, you need to acknowledge and celebrate it.

In his book *Enlightened Leadership*, Doug Krug talks about a version of this practice, called DNA. To get more of what you want, use DNA:

- Define what you want.

- Notice it when you get it.

- Acknowledge/celebrate it.

You need to make sure that when you ask for commitments, you ask for a "yes" or "no." Listen closely for the "yes, but . . ." which you know is another way of saying "no" to a commitment. Also, use requests and offers. What would it take for someone to make a commitment in a particular situation? What could you offer to do to help someone make that commitment? What declarations or assertions do you need to make? What is the effective conversation that you need to have? How do you ask effective questions and how do you actively listen? You need to make sure you listen to understand.

You have to really listen to the other person to understand where he or she is coming from and to understand what may be preventing this person from being able to make a commitment.

You also need to pay attention to the mindset. Is the mindset one of leadership? Is the mindset one of management or administration? We encounter this when we come into meetings. Sometimes we encounter this in meetings when we are with the members of the C-suite. When I go into a meeting in our organization, particularly if someone from the C-suite is there, I am always mindful of the work I am being asked to do in the meeting. I don't go to any meeting just to show up or to be there accidentally. I need to understand the work that is to be accomplished. Am I there just to receive information from a particular person? Am I working with others on a problem that will require management, supervision, or responsibility on my part? Or am I being asked to be in the conversation as a leader to look for possibilities? I need to make sure my mindset is matching the mindset and the work in the room.

If I'm being asked to be part of a group where information is being reported to me, I'm being updated. If I start asking meticulous questions to understand every detail, I'm not paying attention to the mindset in the room. Or, if I'm being asked to be a leader in a meeting, to look for the possibilities, and I start reacting in a very detailed sense, I can easily be perceived to be micromanaging. I need to make sure my mindset in the meeting matches the mindset in the room.

This is a very effective tool when working with members of the C-suite. They are your leaders. You want to hear their leadership story. You need to make sure that when you are dealing with senior executives, you establish the common ground. What do you have in common with them, and how can you all work together to address the situation? One way to establish that common ground is to understand the passion of the senior leader. What makes this person tick? What's his or her leadership story? Why does this person do what he or she does? What's important to this person?

You also need to understand what worries senior executives about a particular situation. The more you understand and effectively listen, and the more you actively listen, the closer you can get to what it would take for them to make a commitment. It's important that you pay attention to that.

I encountered this with our senior executives in a few instances. Several years ago, our CEO shared his leadership story; his passion.

He didn't want to be just another executive of a good health system. He wanted to be the chief executive of a great health system. As he explained his leadership story and his passion to us, it became easy for us to engage in the vision he was setting for the organization. It has also become a touchstone for us, in that as we have continued to work on that strategic plan, we always have his leadership story and his passion to come back to. We always have the direction he set for the organization. We know that because we heard his leadership story, and we understood his passion and his "worries."

It's important when dealing with members of your senior executive team that you listen to the voice you are speaking with, that you understand the person you are working with. You also need to make sure you engage in dialogue. Do not be a passive recipient of information; instead, talk about the information, understand and actively listen, ask effective questions, and look for the commitments that can be made. When you or they are unable to make a commitment, you need to make requests and offers so that you can get to the commitment at hand. You need to provoke commitments and accountability.

Another thing to keep in mind about your C-suite is that senior executives usually don't like surprises. It's important that you understand what's important to them and what they like and don't like so that you can make sure you can get to the point of the commitments at hand.

Another effective tool to use in one-on-one conversations and, especially, in groups, is to "stop and reset." I often think of it as a "timeout." In fact, when I'm in a group of people I know, I sometimes make a T with my hands and say, "Stop, timeout." I use the timeout as an opportunity to reset the energy in the room, essentially the tone of the conversation.

It's also effective to assess the energy in the room or conversation. Is everyone engaged and energized, filling the room with positive energy? Or is everyone focused on all the reasons whatever you are discussing won't work—essentially filling the room with negative energy, which can suck the life out of the room (and you!)?

When you are in an accountability conversation, you need to assess the energy level. Positive energy is about what you can do. Negative energy is about what you cannot do. Net backward energy, according to Doug Krug, is where there are more negatives than positives; more about what you can't do than what you can do. Net forward energy, according to Krug, is about what can be done.

Rather than talking about what can't or won't work, you need to talk about possibilities.

You can ask effective questions such as the following:
- What is working?
- What causes it to work?
- What excites you most about the approach?
- What can you adapt to achieve more of what is working?

- What can you add to improve the results?

- What insights will you gain from hearing about what is working?

You need to be able to focus on how you can flip negative energy. You also need to focus on the work at hand. Are you talking about administration of something, or are you talking about leadership work? You need to make sure you are setting the right context for the work that needs to be done and that you are setting the right environment for achieving accountability, for making commitments, and most especially, for keeping commitments.

Here are a couple of examples of how you can gain accountability from your senior executives and how you can work to make and keep commitments.

☑ ACCOUNTABILITY SPOTLIGHT

Suppose your organization isn't achieving the goals it set for itself. You need to make sure you understand what expectations are not being achieved and where the accountability lies. What commitments have been made? When you are not achieving those commitments, you need to make those requests or make offers about what it would take for those commitments to be met.

In your organization, has a physician ever gone to the CEO instead of coming to you with a problem? It's important to understand that the CEO is in a position of focusing on physician relationships, but that the CEO often recognizes he or she is not the person to fix a particular problem or situation. The CEO should bring the feedback/concern to the level of the organization where that problem can be resolved. If you are the person receiving that information from the CEO, the CEO comes to you and says, "Dr. X is concerned about something, and he brought this concern to me . . ."

You want to make sure the CEO can be accountable for results, and that the CEO understands he or she is not the person to get the situation resolved; you are. You want to make sure the CEO understands that you heard the concern, that you commit to the CEO to resolve the problem, and that the CEO knows he or she can count on you to keep the commitment. So, it's important in this situation that you understand the commitment the CEO is asking of you, that you work with the physician to make a commitment to resolve the situation, and that you can hold the physician accountable to achieve the commitment. Also, make sure that you keep the CEO informed on what has been done to address the problem.

When you work with your senior executives, it is important to understand the world in which they live. I often encounter nurse executives who are concerned about other members of the C-suite not understanding the value of nursing in the organization. In that situation, it's important to think about the particular executive and what makes him or her tick.

Say, for example, that the executive in this case is the chief financial officer (CFO). You could tell him or her the nursing story of why nursing is valuable. However, a far more effective way to hold the CFO accountable for the value of nursing is to make sure nursing understands how a CFO defines value. What result would the CFO need to see to understand the value of nursing, the accountability of nursing? You need to have that conversation with the CFO in terms of the CFO's view of the world, and you need to understand from the CFO's perspective how he or she defines "value" by making requests or offers regarding how you can get the CFO to understand the value of nursing and the commitments nursing can make.

One of the ways we do that in my organization is to make sure nursing leaders are good stewards of the organization's financial resources. This means our nurse leaders need to be able to talk in terms of the financial value of nursing. We talk in terms of productivity and overall performance. We need to use the language our financial colleagues use and make commitments in the context of that language. We need to make sure we make commitments to results—results that are definable, measurable, and time-limited.

In our organization, we have a monthly bed meeting. This meeting includes all nursing directors and managers, as well as our financial partners (accounting and budgeting). Each month, the managers explain their unit's performance and predict their financial performance for the month.

Our financial partners present actual performance by unit for the previous month. If actual financial performance is not what the manager had predicted, the manager presents the plan to correct the unit's performance.

Our financial partners also bring information about trends experienced by the whole organization, resources outside the organization to assist managers, and so forth. We have tackled volume, productivity, and staffing challenges in these meetings.

As a result, we have been very effective in impressing upon our financial partners the value of nursing because we have defined that value in terms that the financial partners can relate to. In addition, our financial partners have successfully shared accountability for the value of nursing with the nursing division.

To hold senior executives accountable, it comes down to the language you use and the situation you create, making sure the results you want are definable, measurable, and time-limited. Be sure you are actively listening. Understand the "voice you are speaking into." Use the DNA tool: Define what you want, notice it when you get it, and then acknowledge it and celebrate it when you see it.

CONTINUING EDUCATION INSTRUCTIONAL GUIDE

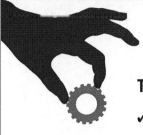

Target Audience

✓ Nurse Managers

✓ Chief Nursing Officers

✓ Chief Nurse Executive

✓ Directors of Nursing

✓ VPs of Nursing

✓ VPs of Patient Care Services

✓ Staff Development Specialists

✓ Directors of Education

✓ Staff Educators

✓ Staff nurses

Statement of Need

A book for nurse managers and nurse leaders featuring practical strategies about how to hold nurses accountable, and also how to practice personal accountability and accountability within multidisciplinary work relationships. The book discusses how nurse managers can focus on changing their culture and creating an environment where nurses are held accountable for all their actions, covering everything from being up-to-date on the latest policies and procedures, to making staff meetings productive events, to practicing excellent patient care. It includes a CD-ROM containing the book's useful tools and training material. (This activity is intended for individual use only.)

Educational Objectives

Upon completion of this activity, participants should be able to:

- Differentiate between responsibility and accountability

- Describe how accountability is demonstrated

- Explain why accountability is important in the nursing profession

- List the six tools in accountability

- Explain the six tools for holding oneself and others accountable

- Identify your personal level of accountability

- Examine your personal communication style

- Describe how to use accountability language and behavior

- Discuss how managers can set accountability expectations

- Describe how to hold staff accountable in a variety of work settings and situations

- Examine how to promote accountability among peers

- Discuss conversation techniques for holding peers accountable

- Assess the level of accountability of your manager or supervisor

- Determine methods to promote accountability from your manager or supervisor

- Examine accountability challenges nurses face with physicians

- Determine how to define expectations

- Explain how to set commitments

- List words to use when interacting with physicians

- List effective words to use with C-suite members

- Describe how to establish common group with C-suite members

- Discuss how your communication style enables C-suite accountability

Faculty

Eileen Lavin Dohmann, RN, MBA, NEA-BC, is vice president of nursing at Mary Washington Hospital in Fredericksburg, VA. She is responsible for nursing care and services as well as operational oversight for MW Home Health and Hospice and The Cancer Center of Virginia.

Nursing Contact Hours

HCPro, Inc. is accredited as a provider of continuing nursing education by the American Nurses Credentialing Center Commission on Accreditation.

This educational activity for 3 nursing contact hours is provided by HCPro, Inc.

Disclosure Statements

HCPro Inc. has confirmed that none of the faculty or contributors have any relevant financial relationships to disclose related to the content of this educational activity.

Instructions

In order to be eligible to receive your nursing contact hours or physician continuing education credits for this activity, you are required to do the following:

1. Read the book *Accountability in Nursing: Six Strategies to Build and Maintain a Culture of Commitment*

2. Complete the exam and receive a passing score of 80%

3. Complete the evaluation

4. Provide your contact information on the exam and evaluation

5. Submit exam and evaluation to HCPro, Inc.

Continuing Education Instructional Guide

Please provide all of the information requested above and mail or fax your completed exam, program evaluation, and contact information to:

> HCPro, Inc.
> Attn: Continuing Education Manager
> P.O. Box 1168
> Marblehead, MA 01945
> Fax: 781/639-2982

NOTE: This book and associated exam are intended for individual use only. If you would like to provide this continuing education exam to other members of your nursing or physician staff, please contact our customer service department at 877/727-1728 to place your order. The exam fee schedule is as follows:

Exam Quantity	Fee
1	$0
2 – 25	$15 per person
26 – 50	$12 per person
51 – 100	$8 per person
101+	$5 per person

CONTINUING EDUCATION EXAM

Name: _____

Title: _____

Facility name: _____

Address: _____

Address: _____

City: _____State: _____ ZIP: _____

Phone number: _____ Fax number: _____

E-mail: _____

Date completed: _____

1. Which of the following statements correctly differentiates accountability from responsibility?

   a. Accountability is a commitment to others to deliver and account for a result by a date, while responsibility pertains to the results to be delivered

   b. Accountability is a commitment to others to deliver and account for a result by a date, while responsibility is authority over things that respond to one's direction

   c. Accountability is authority over things that respond to one's direction, while responsibility is a commitment to others to deliver and account for a result by a date

   d. Accountability is authority over things that respond to one's direction, while responsibility is about things that respond to others

2. Which of the following tools to accountability can nurses use to set the scene for the behavior they want?

    a. Flip negative energy

    b. Active listening

    c. Stop and reset

    d. Framing

3. An accountability culture is important in the nursing profession because:

    a. It enhances nurse–physician collaboration

    b. It decreases medication errors

    c. It reduces staff conflict

    d. It promotes learning, performing, and improving

4. In reference to the "call for the results you want" step to create a culture of accountability, what should nurses do first to involve others in making commitments?

    a. Practice active listening skills

    b. Communicate honestly

    c. Practice accountability language

    d. Define what they want the person to commit to

5. Which of the steps to accountability is the crucial point at which people either make the commitment or don't?

    a. Hear the yes or no

    b. Net forward energy

    c. Flip negative energy

    d. Stop and reset

6. Which of the following questions can nurses ask to identify their personal level of accountability?

    a. Do you usually understand what it expected of you?

    b. Do you often complete tasks that weren't assigned to you?

    c. Do you commit to things that are realistic?

    d. Do you commit to things that are unrealistic?

7. Nurses examining their personal communication style should consider how:

    a. Often they consult their manager for help

    b. Effectively they communicate

    c. Much nursing experience they have

    d. How competent they are in their role

8. How can nurses move forward and practice accountability when others try to avoid commitments and energy turns negative?

    a. Discussing nurses' responsibilities regularly

    b. Discussing what should not be done

    c. Focusing on what can be done

    d. Focusing on what is holding staff back from being accountable

9. How can nurse managers set a clear expectation of accountability in staff members?

    a. Requiring staff to commit to several responsibilities early on

    b. Making staff pay the consequences for being accountable

    c. Communicating to staff that they should know what is expected of them

    d. Avoiding making assumptions that staff members know what is expected of them

10. What can nurse managers ask to hold a staff member accountable after discussing his or her responsibilities?

    a. For the staff nurse to demonstrate his or her commitment

    b. For the staff nurse to discuss what he or she finds dull about the policy

    c. For the staff nurse to tell them what he or she hears

    d. For the staff nurse to sign a contract

11. How can nurses use accountability language to receive a solid commitment from peers when discussing new goals?

    a. Discuss their facility's mission statement and staff's job descriptions

    b. Describe the importance of having a team approach when practicing accountability

    c. Require each nurse to practice accountability

    d. Ask questions about what each nurse is committing to receive defined, measureable, time-limited responses

12. How can nurses use accountability language to increase others' commitments?

    a. Accepting others' negativity and allowing them to make the commitment on their own

    b. Practicing active listening, starting with statements such as "I hear you are frustrated"

    c. Using accountable behavior every day

    d. Communicating directly and respectfully

13. Nurses assessing the level of accountability of their manager or supervisor should request a desired commitment from him or her and _____ if they don't receive the commitment they want.

    a. Consult another member of management
    b. Disregard it
    c. Achieve it themselves
    d. Offer to help achieve it

14. If nurses are in an encounter with their manager and are not hearing accountability, they should _____ to help create a culture of accountability.

    a. Ask other staff members to reiterate their message to that person
    b. Strongly voice their opinion, regardless of potential resulting conflict
    c. Approach another member of management to discuss the matter
    d. Stop the conversation and reset it

15. Which of the following tools can nurses use to find an acceptable solution and obtain a commitment from a busy physician?

    a. Hear the yes or no
    b. Net forward energy
    c. Flip negative energy
    d. Accountability language

16. Which of the following factors may lead to accountability challenges nurses face with physicians?

    a. Nurses' communication styles
    b. Nurses' behaviors
    c. Physicians' communication styles and level of comfort with group thinking
    d. Physicians' behaviors

17. Nurses interacting with physicians should refer to Doug Krug's practice of "DNA," which states to:

    a. Define what you need, notice when you get it, and acknowledge and celebrate it

    b. Define what you want, notice when you get it, and acknowledge and celebrate it

    c. Deliver what is needed and acknowledge and celebrate it

    d. Discuss what you need, notice when you get it, and acknowledge and celebrate it

18. Nurses can create an order set or a protocol with physicians by working with them to define:

    a. A process to see the possibilities and asking what it would take for them to make a commitment to participate in developing and following the order set/protocol

    b. What nurses should do

    c. A process they will follow

    d. What nurses will commit to

19. Which of the following are effective questions nurses can use to achieve accountability from C-suite members during a proposal?

    a. Why wouldn't this be beneficial?

    b. What ways would this contribute to our goals?

    c. Why won't this work?

    d. What is wrong with this proposal?

20. Nurses can establish common ground with C-suite members by:

    a. Understanding the role of the frontline staff nurse

    b. Understanding the role of the senior leader

    c. Understanding the passion of the frontline staff nurse

    d. Understanding the passion of the senior leader

21. Nurses can effectively enable C-suite accountability using a communication style in which they:

    a. Discuss faults of current policies and procedures and measures C-suite needs to take to correct them

    b. Express the needs of patients and how this relates to C-suite accountability

    c. Understand what's important to C-suite members so that they can get to the point of the commitments at hand

    d. Discuss what's important to the entire facility so all hospital staff can be accountable

CONTINUING EDUCATION EVALUATION

Name: _____

Title: _____

Facility Name: _____

Address: _____

Address: _____

City: _____ State: _____ Zip: _____

Phone Number: _____ Fax Number: _____

E-mail: _____

1. This activity met the learning objectives stated:
   ❏ Strongly Agree ❏ Agree ❏ Disagree ❏ Strongly Disagree

2. Objectives were related to the overall purpose/goal of the activity:
   ❏ Strongly Agree ❏ Agree ❏ Disagree ❏ Strongly Disagree

3. This activity was related to my continuing education needs:
   ❏ Strongly Agree ❏ Agree ❏ Disagree ❏ Strongly Disagree

4. The exam for the activity was an accurate test of the knowledge gained:
   ❏ Strongly Agree ❏ Agree ❏ Disagree ❏ Strongly Disagree

5. The activity avoided commercial bias or influence:
   ❏ Strongly Agree ❏ Agree ❏ Disagree ❏ Strongly Disagree

6. This activity met my expectations:
   ❏ Strongly   Agree ❏   ❏ Agree   ❏ Disagree   ❏ Strongly Disagree

7. Will this activity enhance your professional practice?
   ❏ Yes   ❏ No

8. The format was an appropriate method for delivery of the content for this activity:
   ❏ Strongly   Agree ❏   ❏ Agree   ❏ Disagree   ❏ Strongly Disagree

10. If you have any comments on this activity please note them here:

   _____

   _____

   _____

   _____

11. How much time did it take for you to complete this activity?

   _____

Thank you for completing this evaluation of our continuing education activity!

Return completed form to:

HCPro, Inc. • Attn: Continuing Education Manager • P.O. Box 1168, Marblehead, MA 01945
• Tel 877/727-1728 • Fax 781/639-2982

FREE HEALTHCARE COMPLIANCE AND MANAGEMENT RESOURCES!

Need to control expenses, yet stay current with critical issues?

Get timely help with FREE e-mail newsletters from HCPro, Inc., the leader in healthcare compliance education. Offering numerous free electronic publications covering a wide variety of essential topics, you'll find just the right e-newsletter to help you stay current, informed, and effective. All you have to do is sign up!

With your FREE subscriptions, you'll also receive the following:

- Timely information to be read when convenient with your
- Expe...
- Focu...
- Tips

And here's ... n— just a com... gh your daily chall...

It's easy. V... etters/ to register fo... nd let us do the rest.

⊢HCPro | Insight for healthcare compliance and management